MW01502947

Ask Dr. Cory

Cory SerVaas, M.D.

THOMAS NELSON PUBLISHERS

Nashville

Copyright © 1988 by Cory SerVaas, M.D.

All rights reserved. Written permission must be secured from the publisher to use or reproduce any part of this book, except for brief quotations in critical reviews or articles.

Published in Nashville, Tennessee, by Thomas Nelson, Inc., and distributed in Canada by Lawson Falle, Ltd., Cambridge, Ontario.

Printed in the United States of America.

Library of Congress Cataloging-in-Publication Data

SerVaas, Cory.
  Ask Dr. Cory.

  Includes index.
  1. Medicine, Popular. I. Title. II. Title: Ask
Doctor Cory.
RC82.S44 1988   610   88-5212
ISBN 0-8407-7629-2

1 2 3 4 5 6—92 91 90 89 88

CONTENTS

Acknowledgments

We thank the many *Saturday Evening Post* readers for their active involvement, which in turn prompted this book.

We are indebted to Elizabeth Peterson, M.D., Elizabeth Terry, R.N., C.P.N.P., and to Susan Salmon, assistant managing editor at Thomas Nelson Publishers, for their dedicated work in editing our manuscript.

Preface

We hope that some day every medical college in the country will have, along with its departments of OB/GYN, surgery, dermatology, and other specialties, a separate department of prevention. The students in this department would be required to work on preventing disease rather than treating it.

My mentor, Dr. Denis Burkitt (the British medical missionary in Africa who discovered the wonders of fiber in the diet as well as Burkitt's lymphoma, the first cancer thought to be caused by a virus), once illustrated the need for prevention with a cartoon. Many doctors in white jackets carrying pails and mops were mopping up water flooding from a huge sink with a defective faucet. The white-jacketed specialists had all the latest mopping and sponging devices to clean the floor, but there were no swarms of professionals trying to prevent the faucet from flooding. He likened this to the surgeons and internists who are experts in the most recent techniques of handling diseases with drugs and surgery—*after* the damage has been done.

So it is that today's mop-up goes—our experts continue to improve in wielding their mops, and "mop manufacturers" come up with ever more ingenious equipment. But we feel that more dedicated young doctors should be taking a residency in *prevention* to fill well-people's clinics that should be established in America.

Frequently I hear the public complain, "Doctors aren't interested in prevention." I'd like to come to the defense of my colleagues and explain that it is almost impossible for a physician to devote his attention to well people when he has the pressure of helping the sick or the injured. No matter how much resolve I have to stick to prevention, I still get the urge to jump ship and start treating patients and looking for cures.

I just came from seeing a young man, for example, who came to our offices because he had AIDS. He was a handsome, all-American-looking fellow, dying in his twenties. Any doctor with a molecule of compassion would have to start combing his mind for some way to help such a lad.

Physicians are gratified when they see they are helping someone who seeks them out. They are more reluctant to come down hard on smoking cessation or diet change with a patient who has yet to become ill and doesn't want to hear about reform.

And then, a small, practical matter: A physician must make a living for his family, but if he practices prevention only, he will have a hard time knowing which of the patients he has helped avoid a disastrous health problem. How does he bill his well patients who did not go on to get emphysema from smoking, heart disease from a high-fat diet, colon cancer from a low-fiber/high-fat diet, or esophageal cancer from smoking and drinking? People expect to pay for medicines and surgeries; paying for prevention needs to be established for young specialists entering this field.

I was blessed with the undeserved good fortune of a patentable idea early in life and as a result was financially able to go to medical school, while juggling time for a husband and five active, robust children. It was easy for me to choose prevention because I never intended to accept a fee for my medical services. But most doctors need to make a living and haven't had an unusual happenstance to give them the luxury of working at medicine as a labor of love.

Through the Saturday Evening Post Society, I have been able to commit even more resources to prevention. Years before the National Cancer Institute and the Kellogg Company took up the fiber crusade, we introduced our members to the use of wheat bran, a valuable source of insoluble fiber than can lessen the risk of colon cancer and help to prevent diverticulitis, constipation, and other health problems.

We persuaded our Society members to use oat bran for lowering the dangerous LDL cholesterol, which so often portends a heart attack.

We passed along the findings of Dr. James Anderson of the University of Kentucky, who convinced us that the soluble fiber in oats and beans helps to lessen the amount of insulin needed by maturity-onset type II diabetics.

We discovered Dr. Christian Chaussy in Munich, Germany, shortly after he had successfully pulverized his thirteenth kidney stone with his amazing lithotripter. We pioneered the introduction of America's first lithotripter and, through all of this, gave birth to our Kidney Stone Formers Club, from which our rapidly growing Colitis Club is an offshoot.

We took high-lysine corn to Ethiopia and with it the concept of providing more of this essential amino acid for the prevention of kwashiorkor in African toddlers. We also sent seed corn, along with videotaped instructions about why and how to plant it, to Ethiopia and Zimbabwe. Dr. Norman Bourlaug has since been sent by the Rockefeller Foundation to impoverished areas in South America to teach farmers the nutritional value of high-lysine corn for humans, particularly for children.

We are currently campaigning to Snuff Out Snuff, to restrict smoking to its proper place in the city dump, and to exchange fiber for fat in the American diet.

Our mammogram-awareness crusade is spearheaded by the MAMMOBILE and its expert staff, who drive into districts to give mammograms to women who won't go to have this vital breast-cancer-prevention procedure done.

We've been able to influence people to have sigmoidoscopies because they have skin tags. Even though the jury is still out on whether or not people with skin tags have a significantly greater incidence of colon cancer, we do know that a routine sigmoidoscopy, such as President Reagan had, is a good colon-cancer-early-detection measure. Our readers have reported early cancers detected by the sigmoidoscopy, as well as by tests for hidden blood in the stool.

After eight months of sending out our AIDS MOBILE, we have given free, voluntary AIDS tests with counseling to 1,503 persons. From these tests we have identified 31 unsuspecting AIDS-antibody-positive individuals and have given them our list of 23 things to do. For those who already have AIDS, ADC (AIDS dementia complex), or ARC (AIDS-related complex), following these procedures may lengthen the life span considerably. (See page 00.) Furthermore, by following the precautions on the list, they will avoid unwittingly giving AIDS to the ones they love.

Through the years, The Saturday Evening Post Society has responded to people of all ages through *The Saturday Evening Post, Children's Digest, Jack and Jill, Humpty Dumpty,* CBN's "LifeCare Digest," and the *Medical Update* newsletter in an attempt to provide the most up-to-date information on health, nutrition, and fitness, as well as the most recent medical discoveries and developments. A compilation of answers to our readers' most-asked questions, *Ask Dr. Cory* is another step toward our goal of prevention. This book is one more way for us to instill in readers across the country our concern that they pursue the best possible means of keeping themselves healthy now to prevent unnecessary health problems later and to ensure future years of wellness.

The best preventive medicine you can follow is to find a doctor who is well recommended and with whom you are comfortable. Then have an annual physical examination, even if you feel well. Between exams, see your doctor any time you have a health concern. Advice from this book or any other medical book should not prevent you from consulting your own doctor.

Cory SerVaas, M.D.

AIDS: Diagnosis and Prevention

Never has such a dangerous health threat come upon us as suddenly as AIDS, about which little was known a decade ago. And never has a health problem involved so many controversial issues. In retrospect, when knowledge of the disease was first revealed, we didn't act fast enough to prevent the spread.

But much has been learned in a relatively short time. New drugs for pneumocystic pneumonia are keeping AIDS patients alive longer. AZT has shown promise for some. Medical researchers are concentrating on how to prevent the estimated one and one half million AIDS-antibody-positive individuals, who have already been infected, from developing AIDS. Meanwhile, diverse groups such as public-health officers, the general public, and legislators are pondering how to prevent the infected from spreading the sexually transmitted virus.

The following questions seem to be most prevalent in the minds of the public, particularly the readers of *The Saturday Evening Post*.

Q   What causes AIDS?

A   Acquired immunodeficiency syndrome (AIDS) is a serious disease caused by the human immunodeficiency virus (HIV) that reduces the body's ability to fight infection. The people who suffer from AIDS become susceptible to various illnesses, some of which are rare in people whose immune systems function normally. Two such uncommon diseases are *Pneumocystis carinii* pneumonia, a lung infection caused by a protozoa, and

Kaposi's sarcoma, a rare form of cancer of the blood-vessel walls. Tuberculosis, histoplasmosis, lymphomas, and brain diseases are also frequently diagnosed in AIDS patients.

AIDS dementia complex (ADC) is a new AIDS classification. Dr. Richard Price at the Memorial Sloan-Kettering Cancer Center reported that 25 percent of the AIDS victims he has seen showed symptoms of dementia (mental illness) before having any physical complaints. For 9 percent of his patients, AIDS dementia complex (ADC) was the only serious clinical manifestation of HIV infection (AIDS) before death.

Q   I have heard of something called the HIV-antibody test. What is this?

A   When a person is infected by a virus, the body's white blood cells normally begin to fight the infection by producing substances called antibodies. The presence of antibodies, therefore, can indicate whether or not a person has been infected with a virus. Research has shown that the antibodies to HIV are almost always found in the blood of persons who have AIDS or AIDS-related complex or in persons who have been infected with the virus and continue to carry it. However, a negative antibody test does not guarantee that a person is free of the virus, especially if he or she is a member of a group at increased risk of contracting AIDS. If exposure to the virus was recent, antibodies may not have had time to develop.

Q   What does a "negative" test mean?

A   "Negative" test usually signifies that the person tested is free from infection, but not always. It is a test for antibodies. Research indicates that most people will produce antibodies within six months after infection, but a few persons may take twelve to eighteen months to develop antibodies. High-risk individuals with negative test results should have a repeat test several months after the initial test. Persons continuing with high-risk activities should not consider a negative test anything more than a negative result at that point in time.

Q   I read in our local newspaper that since 1985, every pint of blood has been tested by our local Red Cross before it is used for transfusions, so blood is now safe. If the blood bank tests blood to make sure it doesn't have the AIDS virus, can't we be tested when we give blood? I'm not in any high-risk group, but I'm not sure about my ex-husband and would like to know if the blood bank would call me if I came up positive.

A   Quite honestly, no *guarantee* can be made that "blood is now safe" or that the AIDS-antibody screening test used at the blood banks has screened out the virus completely. Persons differ in the way their bodies respond to a virus. Some develop antibodies quickly; some take much longer; there is even the rare individual who doesn't develop antibodies to some viruses. So, you must never go to a blood bank to donate blood if you think you are at even a slight risk. Instead, go to an alternative testing site where testing and counseling are available. The CDC recommends waiting for three months after a suspected exposure before going to be tested. After three months, they believe most people will have had time to develop antibodies to the AIDS virus. Blood banks do have a notification procedure for donors with AIDS-antibody positive blood. The positive blood would, of course, be destroyed.

Q   How would I know if I needed to be tested for AIDS?

A   Anyone who can be included in one of the following groups should be tested for AIDS:

- Sexually active homosexual and bisexual men
- Present and past IV drug users
- Heterosexuals who have had multiple sex partners
- Hemophiliacs
- People who have had blood transfusions
- People who have had organ transplants or donor artificial insemination since 1975
- Sex partners to any of the above
- Infants born to parents at risk

If you are not in a high-risk group, if you haven't had a blood transfusion, and if you know you haven't exposed yourself to the virus, there is no need to be tested. If you know you are safe, you should consider donating your blood for others.

Q   I've heard that some people don't donate blood because they are afraid they can get AIDS by giving blood at a blood bank. Does this ever happen?

A   No, you cannot get AIDS by donating blood. Needles for drawing blood are never reused; they are discarded. In fact, should a medical professional attempt to draw blood from your arm and fail to reach a vein with the needle, he or she will discard the original needle and use a new one when trying again in your other arm. It is perfectly safe to donate blood, and all persons who are in good health and who are sure they've not been exposed to AIDS *should* give blood regularly. Only 5 percent of those able to give blood do so. The need is great.

Q   I understand that all blood donated at blood banks today is tested for the AIDS virus. Does this mean that the blood we receive in a blood transfusion is guaranteed to be safe?

A   No, unfortunately, it can't be guaranteed. *Most* of the blood is safe, but there remains the very small risk that some infected blood can slip through. The AIDS antibody may not develop in the blood until several months after the person has been infected with the virus. So a person who has been recently infected with AIDS may pass the screening test, give blood, and unknowingly contaminate the supply.

When this occurs, painstaking and time-consuming efforts are required to trace the bad blood from recipient to donor. The task becomes increasingly complicated when a patient who tests positive for AIDS has received blood from multiple donors. Such was the case in Indiana when a critically ill patient was given blood transfusions from 175 donors. Because this blood was given after mandatory screening tests were in effect, all units were believed to be safe. However, infectious blood had apparently passed through the window during the antibody screening test at the blood bank. (The "window" refers to the period when the donor is infectious but his antibodies have not yet developed.)

The patient recovered from the original illness but later tested positive for the AIDS virus. The diagnosis touched off an intensive search campaign by the regional blood center. An attempt was made to locate all 175 donors who would be urged to undergo another AIDS test. In this tragic event, however, 10 of the 175 donors had left no forwarding addresses at the post office and could not be notified. Those who were retested were all negative, and the donor who gave the infected blood was never located.

When people are found to be HIV positive after receiving blood, scientific investigators always consider that the person might have been HIV positive before the questionable blood was received. The Saturday Evening Post Society advises its members to ask their doctors for an AIDS test before any surgery that may require a blood transfusion. This inexpensive baseline test showing negative might then prevent conjecture by blood banks that perhaps it wasn't the transfusion but a prior high-risk life style that had caused the viral antibody seroconversion.

Q   How can we help to make the blood bank supply safer?

A   First, you can *give* blood if you are in good health and certain you have not been exposed to AIDS.

Second, you can help to educate people concerning the risk involved when persons who have been recently exposed to AIDS give blood. AIDS is apparently a slow-developing virus and not everyone develops antibodies to the virus in the same length of time. Because antibodies can take longer to show up in the blood than previously thought, the blood bank is unable to positively detect *all* AIDS carriers with the antibody test.

Third, you can contact legislators and ask them to pass a law making it possible to trace blood donors through their Social Security numbers. The law should also require all blood donors to agree to come back for retesting if their blood was included in the group of units from which a person contracted AIDS. At present it isn't possible for blood banks to require this retesting.

No one needs to fear that the results of antibody testing done at the blood bank will be made public. Physicians supervising blood banks are trained to keep all health information concerning patients confidential.

We hope that the public will persevere until the blood supply can be guaranteed free from AIDS.

Q   I know that I am to have major surgery later this year and that I will require several units of blood. Is there any way I can make sure that a truly safe supply of blood will be available for me when I need it?

A   There are several options. You may be able to donate your own blood in advance and have it stored until you need it. This is called autologous donation, or pre-donation. If you do not use your predonated blood, you can give it to the blood bank after your surgery.

AIDS is not the only reason for autologous blood donation. A type of hepatitis called non-A, non-B hepatitis may be present in donated blood and cannot be screened out by any test now available. By planning ahead and providing a supply of your own blood, you can protect yourself from any risk of exposure. You can't give yourself something you don't already have.

If you are planning to undergo surgery in the future, you'll need to give your doctor plenty of time to arrange for autologous transfusion. Your doctor will check your hematocrit level to see if you are anemic. Your doctor might choose to prescribe an iron supplement because if your hematocrit level falls below 34 percent, you will not be able to predonate.

Another alternative to ensure that you have a safe supply of blood is to have the surgeons arrange to salvage the blood lost during surgery. The blood is "washed" and transfused back into the patient. This can't be done for some surgeries, however.

Directed donations are more difficult to arrange than autologous donations. *Directed* means a relative or friend donates blood for you. As with predonations, if the directed donation isn't needed, it can be given to the blood bank.

When people travel in African countries where the blood supply is hazardous, they are advised to take plasma expanders and blood substitutes with them or travel with a "buddy" of the same blood type who can donate in an emergency. Plasma expanders can sometimes be used to prevent or postpone the need for a transfusion of whole blood.

Q   How long can blood be kept after it is donated?

A   Unfrozen blood stored in the refrigerator can be kept for up to six weeks. Frozen blood can be kept almost indefinitely.

Q   What if I am caught in an emergency situation and the only blood available is frozen?

A   It takes about 90 minutes to thaw and prepare frozen blood. Plasma expanders may be used for a patient during that interim.

Q   How do you know whether or not you will need a blood transfusion before surgery?

A   If you are scheduled for elective surgery, you should ask your doctor about the possibility of a blood transfusion. If he answers that a transfusion is possible, you should consider predonating your own blood.

Dr. Pearl T.C.Y. Toy and her colleagues completed a national multicenter study recently published in the *New England Journal of Medicine* in which they reported on 4,996 patients undergoing elective surgery at eighteen hospitals: "Cross-matched blood was ordered for 1,287 patients (26 percent), and of these, 590 (46 percent) were considered eligible for predepositing blood. Only 5 percent (32) of the eligible patients actually predeposited blood, indicating that predonation is not widely used."

The authors concluded: "Greater use of predonation would not only reduce the demand on the blood supply by decreasing the need for homologous (outside donor) transfusion, but would probably also reduce the risk of hepatitis and other transfusion-associated illnesses."

(If you would like additional information about this subject, you may write to: Safe Blood, P.O. Box 567, Indianapolis, IN 46202.)

Q I am pregnant and am scheduled to have a Caesarean section. My doctor says I may need blood. My husband said he would like to give blood and have it stored for me. Is this ever done?

A Yes, you can arrange for compatible blood to be stored for you. Your question involves a subject very close to my heart. Our son, Eric, and his lovely wife, Marcia, who is the mother of their three beautiful daughters, are expecting triplets very soon. Marcia will require a C-section because, she says, "They are packed in like sardines and the bottom baby is in a breech position."

Eric can't donate blood for her because their blood types are incompatible. Her brother, Mark, is compatible and has predonated blood which is now frozen so there will be blood in an emergency. Some argue that a directed donor may not necessarily be a safe donor, but in Mark's case, he has been giving blood regularly for the past several years. If the triplets are delivered prematurely, they may also need blood transfusions. Eric, the babies' father (also a regular blood donor), will be available to donate blood in the event he is the proper blood type for the triplets. Thus, neither Marcia nor the babies will have to risk a hepatitis B or AIDS virus being transmitted.

Dr. William J. Ledger, a prominent OB/GYN and the chairman of the obstetrics department at the New York Hospital-Cornell Medical Center, discussed this subject:

Autologous (self-donated) blood transfusions can be offered as a safe alternative in obstetrical patients. This has been accomplished without incident at the New York Hospital-Cornell Medical Center.

A potentially controversial additional recommendation is donation of blood by spouses of these women if they have a compatible blood group and type. There are many arguments against this (e.g., these donors are not

safer, it unnecessarily increases the work load, there is no real advantage to the patient). These arguments have a familiar ring and are similar to initial discussions about fathers being present in the labor and delivery room. The arguments against this were that the presence of the fathers had no benefit and that it complicated the delivery of medical care. The actual experience in obstetrics has been the opposite. It has been beneficial to everyone, and today's fathers are an integral part of the labor and birthing process. If a responsible couple have compatible blood groups and Rh types, the husbands should be able to donate blood for wives who need gynecologic or obstetrical surgical care.

Dr. Ledger points out, "The arguments for screening all pregnant women are rapidly becoming stronger as the number of HIV-positive individuals in the community increases."

Q   Are just IV drug abusers at risk for AIDS? What about people who are cocaine addicts but don't "shoot up"?

A   You ask an important question. Non-IV drug users also have a high incidence of AIDS because abuse of drugs, alcohol, and tobacco lowers a person's immunity. These drug addicts often engage in prostitution and promiscuous sex.

Q   How often can I donate blood?

A   You can give a pint every eight weeks, up to five times a year.

Q   In addition to the AIDS antibody (ELISA) test, what are some of the other tests that blood banks use to screen donors?

A   Tests for syphilis, hepatitis B antigen, and various liver functions are used by blood banks. There is no available screening test for non-A, non-B hepatitis.

Q   I know that in the past hemophiliacs have been infected with AIDS through blood transfusions and through treatment with a blood-derived product that gives them the clotting agent their blood lacks. Has a way been found to protect hemophiliacs from this risk?

A   Hemophiliacs still receive blood from many different donors, but two safeguards are in place today. The blood comes from screened donors, and the clotting agents from the blood are heat-treated to kill any AIDS virus that might be present.

Q   I've had the AIDS antibody test and the results were negative. I know, however, that I may have been exposed to AIDS a few weeks earlier. What should I do?

A   As a responsible person, you will assume that you may be carrying the AIDS virus, and you should take precautions to protect yourself and others. (See the list of 23 precautions on page 24.)
We know that after a victim has become infected, the antibodies are not immediately detectable. This period of time is the "window," during which the AIDS virus would not be detected in any tests currently being done on donated blood. We called the Centers for Disease Control for updated information about safety in blood screening. We asked, "How long can a person be infectious with the AIDS virus and still not have an antibody concentration high enough to be caught in screening tests?" Charles Schable responded:

It is difficult to say, because it depends on the person's biological response, and it depends on the volume of inoculation. Someone who stuck a (contaminated) nee-

21

dle in himself is going to react differently than someone who got a unit of infected blood.

Plus, a lot of people don't know exactly when they were inoculated. . . . When a male homosexual has had numerous exposures, how does he know who was positive or who was a drug addict sticking a needle in himself every day? How do we know when the exact exposure occurs? So a lot of the data are based on individuals who had received bad blood, if you want to use that term. We know that antibodies can come up very quickly—that is, five to ten weeks. If you test somebody every day, you are obviously going to pick it up very fast, if you know when they were inoculated. But how many people are going to get tested every day? So we at the Centers for Disease Control recommend that if you think you have been exposed, you should go get tested after 120 days. Generally speaking, if you haven't developed antibodies by then, you are not going to—although it is not 100 percent certain.

Q Is it possible for a woman to get AIDS from artificial insemination?

A This has happened in the past, but there are now safeguards in place to prevent it from happening. When the male donor tests negative for AIDS, his semen is frozen and stored. After a year, another blood sample is taken from the donor and tested for AIDS. This procedure allows time for antibodies to develop if the AIDS virus was in his system at the time he gave the semen. Only after this second test proves negative is the semen used for artificial insemination.

Q I keep hearing that we shouldn't do a lot of voluntary testing because of false positives. What is the prevalence of false positives?

A   The Department of Defense has tested in excess of 4 million persons and has recently assessed a false-positive rate of 1 out of 135,000 low-risk individuals (after repetitive ELISA positives and confirmatory Western blot tests). The one false positive could be checked further by studying T cells and by culturing the virus from the blood.

Dr. Judith Johnson, an infectious disease specialist at Indiana University, said:

> I don't want any AIDS-antibody-positive individuals to dismiss their results as being false positive. I fear that patients may deny their high-risk behavior and rationalize away their test results. Most seropositive people, if they review their past history, will be able to find some risk factor. For example, after thinking about a positive AIDS diagnosis, a patient might make a comment like, "Well, I did have surgery in 1980 with blood transfusions." Persons who truly cannot find any risks should talk to their doctor about further tests.

Dr. Brooks Jackson of the St. Paul Red Cross and Minnesota state epidemiologist Dr. Michael Osterholm tested more than 250,000 low-risk patients—blood donors—and found *no* false positives. They found 15 positives, which were confirmed by Western blot tests. Each of the 15 admitted to being high risk. The AIDS virus was actually cultured from the blood of the 13 patients who came in for follow-up blood testing. The fourteenth patient was already symptomatic with AIDS. The fifteenth admitted to high-risk behavior.

The AIDS virus culture takes one month, and the procedure presently costs about $150. But it is expected that this cost will soon drop. The army paid $4.00 per person for the repetitive ELISA tests and confirmatory Western blot tests.

The conclusive results of the Department of Defense and of Drs. Osterholm and Jackson—who will be submitting the results of their research for publication—could lay to rest the head-in-the-sand attitude that fear of false-positive tests should prevent the testing of low-risk populations. Because the test is so accurate, it should become a routine part of physicals for those who believe they have even the slightest risk.

Q Why be tested for the AIDS antibody?

A For anyone with some risk, it is important to know one's AIDS-antibody status. If you should happen to be AIDS-antibody positive, the following precautions might save your life or the life of someone you love.

For those who already have AIDS, ADC (AIDS dementia complex), or ARC (AIDS-related complex), following these procedures may lengthen the lifespan considerably.

1. If you are AIDS-antibody positive, pregnancy may weaken your immune system and bring on AIDS, AIDS-related complex, or AIDS dementia complex. The baby has a 40 to 60 percent chance of having AIDS. In an infected mother, breast milk contains the AIDS virus, so you should avoid breast feeding.
2. Avoid live-virus vaccines, such as those for measles, mumps, rubella, and polio.
3. Get a doctor's recommendations about pneumococcal and flu vaccinations, which are often recommended. These are inactivated, rather than live vaccines.
4. Polio can be contracted by an AIDS-antibody-positive person from oral-polio-vaccine virus excreted in the stool of a vaccinated child or adult. No oral polio (live-virus) vaccine should be given in a household with an AIDS-antibody-positive person.
5. Your doctor will not use immunosuppressive

drugs, such as corticosteroids. Certain anticancer drugs are dangerous for AIDS-positive persons.

6. Don't use aspirin or other painkillers without consulting your doctor. Aspirin is slightly immunosuppressive.

7. Do not use illicit drugs, including marijuana and heroin, as they are immunosuppressive.

8. Encourage your spouse, ex-spouse, and/or sex partner to have the AIDS antibody test.

9. Protect your sex partner by informing him or her of your condition. Condoms improve safety but do not remove all risks.

10. Use your own razor blades, manicure scissors, and toothbrushes—don't share. Don't have your ears pierced or get tatooed.

11. Decontaminate all surfaces that have come in contact with blood by cleaning with household bleach, diluted one part bleach to ten parts water.

12. AIDS-antibody-positive persons should not clean cat litter or bird cages. Cats transmit toxoplasmosis. Birds transmit histoplasmosis and psittacosis. These infections could be quite hazardous to the immune-compromised person.

13. Notify your physician, dentist, and any other medical personnel that you have had a positive antibody test so they can do their best to care for you and to prevent the spread of the virus. You will be watched more closely for infection and treated earlier and more aggressively than someone with a more dependable immune system.

14. Ask your family doctor to help you select a physician who specializes in infectious diseases or immune deficiency to do additional blood tests. Such tests will reveal the condition of your protective T-cells. These specialists are also trained AIDS medical counselors. Further, professional ethics dictate that physicians maintain confidentiality.

15. Ask your doctor about the possibility of taking AZT (an experimental AIDS drug). There is some hope that AZT may be more effective if taken in the early stages of HIV infection.

16. Do not donate blood, plasma, sperm, body organs, or other tissues.

17. Avoid unpasteurized milk, because there is a risk of salmonella, TB, or campylobacter infections, all of which are more serious in an immunosuppressed person. Avoid undercooked meat.

18. It is especially important that AIDS-antibody-positive persons exercise regularly, maintain a proper diet, get adequate rest, and avoid stress to help maintain the immune system.

19. AIDS-antibody-positive individuals need to know that they are at greater risk to have serious consequences from the traveler's diarrhea that tourists jokingly refer to as "Montezuma's Revenge" or "Delhi Belly." If you must visit Third World countries, take bottled water and avoid raw foods.

20. To protect your immune system, do not use alcoholic beverages or use in moderation. Alcohol is immunosuppressive. Abstain from tobacco products. They, too, are immunosuppressive.

21. Assiduously avoid all additional sexually transmitted infections, such as cytomegalovirus, papillomavirus, syphilis, and reinfections with the AIDS virus.

22. Do not visit sick friends at home or in the hospital if they have an infection so that you don't risk getting it.

23. You should carefully consider pros and cons of elective surgical procedures like cosmetic surgery or dental transplants because of higher potential for infection. When undergoing surgery of any kind, discuss with your physician the advantages and disadvantages of protective treatment with antibiotics prior to surgery.

Q What is a "positive" test?

A Because it is possible that multiple exposures to HIV or other agents are required for the development of AIDS, people with positive tests need frequent medical evaluations. Further, people who have positive tests can transmit the virus to someone else, who may develop AIDS and die from it, though the carrier remains well.

Some of the best physicians and scientists in the country are working at breakneck speed to find a cure for AIDS, a vaccine to prevent AIDS, and, most important for the AIDS-antibody-positive individual, a way to prevent carriers from developing ARC (AIDS-related complex), ADC (AIDS dementia complex), or AIDS. Although we do not know how many of today's AIDS-antibody-positive individuals will develop AIDS, we are trying to discover through current research how to delay and possibly prevent AIDS, ARC, or ADC.

Q What does the average American think about AIDS education and testing?

A If *Saturday Evening Post* readers are average Americans, we know what 10,964 average Americans think. This is the number who have currently answered our survey.

When we asked, "Do you believe that children should be taught about AIDS prevention in school," 9,863 said yes; 877 said no; and 224 didn't answer the question.

Of those who said yes, the average age at which they believed a child should be taught about AIDS was 10.

We asked, "Do you believe that hospitals should be required to routinely check all patients who have received blood for the rare possibility of an AIDS-antibody-positive result?" 9,981 answered yes; 781 said no; 202 gave no answer.

We asked, "In your opinion should insurance companies be prohibited from requiring applicants to take an AIDS test as a prerequisite for obtaining insurance?" 2,827 said yes; 6,209 said no; 1,928 said they didn't know.

We asked: "Do you believe that all those who apply for marriage licenses should be tested for AIDS?" 9,883 said yes; 767 said no; 314 gave no answer.

We asked: "Do you believe there should be a law making it mandatory for blood donors to leave their forwarding addresses with the post office or their blood bank when they move or leave town, so that they can be contacted and tested in the rare event that their blood is believed to have caused AIDS in a recipient?" 9,507 said yes; 555 said no; 902 didn't know.

We asked: "What do you believe is the incidence of hepatitis from blood transfusions?" 5,157 said 1 percent; 2,613 said 10 percent; and 856 said 20 percent; 2,338 didn't answer. (The correct answer is 10 percent.)

Q How many HIV positive persons have been discovered by the AIDS MOBILE testing project?

A Currently, 31 persons have been discovered. 1,503 persons have been counseled and tested for the AIDS virus. The 31 persons include a young nursing mother who had transfusions during a Caesarian section, and several young people who had been on drugs years earlier.

Nutrition and Fitness

Thousands of *The Saturday Evening Post* readers write in questions relating to nutrition and fitness. Because of discoveries showing that poor nutrition increases the possibility of cancer, heart conditions, appendicitis, diverticulosis, hemorrhoids, gall bladder complications, and other diseases, we are more concerned than ever about the food we eat. Many of us are establishing high-fiber/high-carbohydrate/low-fat diets, as well as heeding warnings and recommendations by doctors, the National Cancer Institute, and the American Heart Association. The following questions and answers illustrate some of the fundamental principles for healthy eating and fitness.

CHOLESTEROL REDUCTION

Q   My husband has a high cholesterol level. Some diets recommend oatmeal and others recommend oat bran for cholesterol reduction. Which is better?

A   Oatmeal is fine for soluble fiber, but you would have to eat a lot more of it to get the same amount of fiber that you get in a bowl of oat bran. Quaker Oat Bran is available in grocery stores, and Mother's Oat Bran, made by Quaker, is available in health-food stores.

Oat bran contains soluble fiber, which is good for lowering one's risk for a coronary, a stroke, and early senility from clogging cholesterol plaques. Soluble fibers lower the low-density lipoproteins (LDL), the bad cholesterol. In an experiment with students at MIT, those who ate oat muffins made with soluble fibers were said to lower their chances of having heart attacks by 10 percent, as compared with those eating wheat bran muffins.

Wheat bran, however, contains more insoluble fiber, which causes bulk in the stool, prevents constipation, and is believed to help in preventing cancer of the colon.

BOWEL CONTROL

Q   I have been trying to increase my intake of fiber and have tried a variety of bean recipes. The trouble is that these products cause excessive flatulence. Is there any natural remedy or method of preparation that can eliminate this problem?

A   If you will drink at least eight cups of warm water daily, you will have less gas. Although we don't understand why, cold water doesn't relieve flatus as well as warm water. You can also drink citrus tea—a quarter of a lime squeezed into hot water with mint leaves and some prune juice to sweeten and color it. Don't substitute regular tea or coffee for water because they contain caffeine and xanthine, which cause tissues to retain water. Adding baking soda to your beans also causes water retention because of the sodium content. Exercise also helps relieve gas.

Passing gas from the colon is not harmful to your health though most people are embarrassed by the occurrence. It's better to ignore the flatus and eat the beans than to suffer the real problem of a colostomy bag, the result of a refined, fiber-depleted, bland diet.

Q   I have had a constipation problem over the years, and I am allergic to wheat. What fiber can I use to eliminate my constipation and diverticulosis?

A   A recent study has suggested that corn fiber (as found in corn bran) is the best of all fiber grains for alleviating constipation.

VITAMINS AND MINERALS

Q   Do I need a calcium supplement to my diet? I don't like milk and try to avoid the cholesterol in cheeses. Will calcium help to prevent osteoporosis?

A   Research indicates that a woman prior to menopause needs 1000 mg of calcium per day; after menopause, she requires 1400 mg per day. A study at the University of North Carolina has shown that three out of four college-aged women don't get enough calcium in their diets. Other studies have shown that 65 percent of the women and nearly half of the males in their twenties don't consume the minimum daily requirement of calcium.

If your diet is chronically calcium deficient, your body draws calcium from the bones as a defense mechanism, in some instances causing a disease called osteoporosis. Osteoporosis causes bones to become shrunken and brittle. The cervical vertebrae shrink, the neck shortens, and because the leftover skin has nowhere to go, it becomes wrinkled. As the person with osteoporosis shrinks in height, the waistline thickens, and then finally disappears when the rib cage comes to rest on the pelvis.

Adequate calcium intake may help you in other ways. Dr. David McCarron of the University of Oregon reported that the lack of calcium may be a factor in hypertension. And from the Sloan-Kettering Cancer Center, Dr. Martin Lipkin found that calcium supplements of 1,250 mg a day caused significant changes in the lining of the colon of high-cancer-risk patients.

Q   How do I get calcium into my diet?

A   Dairy products, green leafy vegetables, sardines, salmon (with their bones), tofu, and certains nuts are excellent sources of calcium. A high-calcium cereal made with yogurt has also been developed.

A convenient and practical way to meet the daily calcium need is to take calcium supplements. They are inexpensive, and there are many kinds from which to choose. To maximize their effect, calcium supplements should not be taken at the same time as a vitamin/mineral supplement, since the latter may contain zinc, which can inhibit the absorption of calcium. Also, because the body is unable to absorb a day's dosage—approximately 1,000 mg—at one time, it is best to take 500 to 600 mg twice a day, one hour after eating. Remember the following practical points:

1. Note the amount of elemental calcium on the label and select preparations that have calcium carbonate. This substance releases more calcium, weight for weight, than other calcium supplements. If you take calcium carbonate and it causes gas, try calcium citrate instead.

2. Calculate the amount of calcium you usually have in your diet and meet the deficiency with more calcium-containing foods or calcium supplements. Most women will need to supplement with 500 to 750 mg of extra calcium each day. The supplement should be taken two or three times daily to maximize absorption.

3. Beware of the so-called bone-robber, caffeine. As few as two cups of coffee per day can greatly increase the excretion of calcium from the body.

4. Postmenopausal women should speak with their physicians concerning the benefits and risks to supplemental estrogen, which is known for its bone-saving potential.

Q   Do foods lose their vitamin C content if exposed to air or water? How much of the vitamin is lost?

A   Yes. The Idaho potato is an example of a food that loses much of its vitamin C when stored. The potatoes are dug in the fall and kept in storage for many months. After only one month of storage, a potato loses 25 percent of its vitamin C content. If a potato is dug in September, it will lose 50 percent of its vitamin C by Christmas, and 25 percent more by spring.

Q   How does vitamin C help the body?

A   Vitamin C is important in preventing the dangerous breakdown of nitrates and nitrites into carcinogens called nitrosamines. Processed, smoked, and cured meats—including ham, bacon, pastrami, bologna, corned beef, dried beef, sausages, hot dogs, and luncheon meats—are treated with nitrates and nitrites to prevent spoilage. By adding powdered vitamin C to your chipped beef on toast, ham casseroles, beans and franks, and other processed-meat recipes, you can prevent the breakdown of the nitrates. This may be more convenient than having family members take vitamin C in capsule or pill form.

Most physicians agree that vitamin C is imperative for the healing of wounds and bad burns. If you must be hospitalized for any reason and you have been supplementing your diet with a high quantity of vitamin C, be sure you inform your physician. If you require intravenous feedings, the physician will ensure that your IV fluids contain sufficient vitamin C to avoid an abrupt change in your vitamin C intake.

ALCOHOLISM AND VITAMIN B_1

Q   Why are many alcoholics prone to B_1 deficiency?

A   With thirteen million alcoholics in the United States suffering from nutritional deficiencies, alcoholism is the leading cause of nutritional deficiencies in our country. This happens for several reasons. The steady drinker focuses on consuming alcohol, not food. Additionally, alcohol prevents efficient absorption of some nutritional elements. To make matters worse, drinking increases the demand for B vitamins, which are necessary to metabolize the carbohydrates furnished by the alcohol itself.

The vitamin most vulnerable to alcohol is B_1, also known as thiamine. A serious B_1 deficiency can result in Wernicke-Korsakoff's syndrome, a thiamine-deficiency disease that ultimately causes irreversible brain and peripheral nerve damage in alcoholics. At first the alcoholic may experience burning feet, tingling, or the absence of sensation. Later he or she may develop a stumbling gait, personality changes, or double vision. Confusion and forgetfulness of recent events may lead the alcoholic to make up stories to cover for his memory loss—a condition doctors refer to as confabulation. Thiamine deficiency is the predominant reason that alcoholics become psychotic.

Prompt injection of this B vitamin may be life saving for an alcoholic having convulsions. Microscopic examination reveals small hemorrhages in the midbrain and in the cerebral cortex of alcoholics who die in convulsions. In 1952 researchers concluded that Wernicke's encephalopathy is corrected by thiamine alone, except when irreversible brain damage has already occurred. There appears to be a genetic inability of some people to tolerate thiamine deprivation.

Fortunately, thiamine is nontoxic and inexpensive. If you have a heavy drinker in the house, you might consider adding crushed vitamin B_1 to his alcoholic beverages. The B_1 can give him a better appetite, help with digestion, soothe his nerves, make him feel happier, and allow him to better metabolize carbohydrates for more energy. Since most alcoholics don't eat well, they need supplemental thiamine to make up for poor absorption. A multivitamin will help too.

Good food sources of thiamine are whole grains, brewer's yeast, dried beans and peas, leafy vegetables, and cauliflower. Foods containing nitrates, such as bologna, salami, and smoked meats, decrease the availability of thiamine to the body. Thiamine is leached out of boiled foods, but by using the cooking water as stock for soup the thiamine can be retrieved. Because thiamine is water soluble, it is not stored in the body. A daily supply is needed.

Q   I have an iron deficiency. How can I increase my iron intake?

A   Anemia pervades every age group in our culture. As many as 10 percent of the preschool-age children in the United States are iron deficient, the peak incidences occuring among one and two year olds. Irregular dietary habits, rapid growth spurts, and the current predilection for junk foods contribute to iron deficiency in adolescents. Pregnant women need iron supplements, as do elderly people who develop poor eating habits often from apathy or depression.

Beginning in infancy, a person's diet should include sufficient iron. Milk creates an alkaline diet, in which iron is poorly absorbed. Because of the gradual development of an iron deficiency, the body may adapt well and show few symptoms of anemia. Some people, however, experience fatigue, headaches, irritability, tingling of the extremities, and shortness of breath.

You can get much of the iron you need by eating foods such as liver, wheat germ, dried apricots, cashews, and lentils. Depending on your age and gender, you may need an intake of 10 to 30 mg of iron each day. The average American diet provides only about 6 mg of iron in every 1,000 calories.

We only absorb about one-tenth of the iron in the foods we eat. To improve absorption, eat vitamin C (ascorbic acid) along with the foods containing iron. Dark green vegetables, cauliflower, cabbage, tomatoes, cantaloupe, oranges, and strawberries are "C" foods that can be eaten at the same meal as your iron-rich foods.

Another inexpensive way to increase the iron in your diet is to use iron cooking utensils. Cooking acid foods in an iron vessel provides more usable iron in your diet.

Q   My friend had a baby with spina bifida. What can be done to prevent this problem?

A   Spina bifida refers to the failure of the spinal column to close properly during the first three weeks of pregnancy. This defect—occurring in one to two babies out of every thousand—can result in a person's being seriously handicapped for life.

Although the cause of spina bifida is not known for certain, it appears to be multiple environmental and genetic factors. Advances in neurosurgical research and better control of infections with antibiotics have made it possible for an estimated 80 to 95 percent of babies born today with spina bifida to survive and grow to maturity.

British scientists found that women who took a vitamin supplement with folic acid (a B vitamin found in green leafy vegetables) before conception and during the first three weeks of pregnancy had fewer babies with spina bifida than a similar group of women who did not take the vitamins. Some researchers believe that chemicals or drugs that decrease a woman's supply of folic acid can increase her baby's chance of having spina bifida. Avoidance of hyperthermia (increased body temperature, such as from a hot bath) early in pregnancy may also be helpful.

ADDITIVES AND PRESERVATIVES

Q I want to eliminate food additives and preservatives from my diet. What are sulfites? Are they unhealthy?

A Some additives, such as the vitamins that enrich flour and the iodine in table salt, are beneficial. However, others may not be nutritious and could even be dangerous for some individuals. One such substance is sulfite, which is used in most dried fruits—apples, apricots, peaches, pears, bananas—with the exception of golden raisins and prunes. Potato packagers currently use sulfites to keep potatoes from turning brown when peeled; however, a regulation with regard to its use in potato products in pending. Shrimp are usually treated with sulfites, as are most American wines. Commercial apple pies and cocktail mixes, including those made with real lemon or wine, contain sulfite.

Although sulfites are not harmful for most people, they have triggered serious attacks in people who have asthma or who are allergic to the additive. In 1985 the FDA received 150 complaints of reactions to sulfite, and 20 deaths were attributed to the reactions. About three-fourths of the people reporting reactions had a history of asthma. Forty percent of persons registering complaints had eaten raw fruits and vegetables from salad bars before their reactions. Fifteen percent blamed their reactions on wine.

The most common symptom of a sulfite reaction is difficulty in breathing. Other symptoms include difficulty in swallowing, tightening of the chest, nausea, diarrhea, faintness or unconsciousness, abdominal pain, cramps, hives, weakness, headaches, and a blue discoloration of the skin because of poor circulation.

If you think you might be sulfite-sensitive, an allergist can monitor your reactions while you sip graduated doses of sulfite in fruit juices. (Your doses are regulated so you're never at any serious risk.) The allergist tests your pulmonary function by noting any decrease in the amount of air you can exhale. You are considered allergic to sulfites if the amount of air you exhale drops 20 percent in one second. Of course, you can be certain you're allergic if you have a skin reaction.

Various sulfite compounds appear on food product labels: sulfur dioxide, sodium sulfite, sodium and potassium bisulfite, and sodium and potassium metabisulfite. The FDA is considering new regulations on sulfites, and many restaurants and grocers have already voluntarily quit using the additives.

Although the sulfite content of restaurant foods is not indicated on menus, you can test any foods with test strips you can order through the mail. The strips turn red if sulfites are present in the food. We sprinkled sulfur dioxide on a piece of brown, limp lettuce, and the lettuce became bright green and looked edible. We then applied a test strip, which turned red. In spite of our attempts to wash and even rub it off, the sulfite was still there.

Persons sensitive to sulfite need to be alert for sulfites in dried foods and should consider drying their own. Dried foods have the same nutritional value as frozen foods and more than canned foods. Drying food is also economical.

Q   I have ulcerative colitis and have had to eliminate milk from my diet. How can I prepare dishes that require it?

A   Because milk is found in many foods, you may find you want to include it in your diet by taking Lactaid™ or Lactrase™, available without a prescription in drugstores. These products contain an enzyme that makes milk easier to digest. Another alternative to use in cooking is soy milk.

PREVENT HEMORRHOIDS WITH DIET

Q   I've heard high-fiber diets are beneficial in preventing hemorrhoids. How satisfactory are fiber supplements in producing the same effects?

A   The populations of countries where a high-fiber diet is consumed have an extremely low incidence of hemorrhoids. The importance of fiber has been shown since ancient Greece. Hippocrates said, "To the human body it makes a great difference whether the bread be fine or coarse; of wheat with or without the hull."

You may lessen your risk for developing hemorrhoids by adding more bran and whole grains to your diet. For patients whom doctors term noncompliant—that is, they will not be able to change their lifelong eating habits to include enough fiber in their diets—doctors like to recommend products, such as Metamucil or Fiberall, made of ground psyllium seed fiber.

Metamucil and Fiberall come in sugar-free packages and are even made in special fruit flavors, like orange and strawberry. These natural fibers absorb several times their weight in liquid and don't contain chemical stimulants. They provide a safe and effective means of softening the stool and helping to prevent hemorrhoids.

If you travel, Metamucil and Fiberall are easy to find in drugstores and supermarkets everywhere. Since my husband and I travel a lot, not only do we pack a bran pouch, but we also pack a plastic container of wheat berries (whole kernels). We cook wheat berries and keep a jar of them in the refrigerator at all times. On trips we add them to room-service soups, vegetables and rice, and sprinkle them on salads. At home, they make a great breakfast cereal and have a chewy texture that goes well with skim milk and a favorite fruit.

HOSPITAL AND NURSING HOME NUTRITION

Q   During a recent hospital stay my aged aunt became depressed and lethargic, hardly eating any of the food set before her. Instead of her health improving, I felt it deteriorated. Do you have any nutritional suggestions that would have made her trip to the hospital more beneficial?

A   A large number of individuals admitted to a hospital, especially the elderly, are already undernourished, and the problem merely intensifies during their stay because of illness, surgery, and the differences in types of food offered from the patients' usual diet. In 1984 the Nutrition Society conducted a survey that revealed the quality of hospital food to be lower than the quality the average person normally eats. Hospital diets generally have more fat and less fiber than the average person's diet.

Often, hospital patients and nursing-home residents, especially those with orthopedic problems, get little exercise so that they lose their appetite. Yet illness increases the metabolic rate so the patients actually need more food.

Hospitals are becoming more attuned to the nutritional needs of the patients. Hospital dieticians visit "problem" patients to analyze their nutritional needs and ensure adequate nutrition. When alternative means of providing nutrition are necessary, such as feeding with a needle in the vein or a nasalgastric tube that goes through the nostrils into the stomach, patients experience the particular risk of becoming deficient in potassium, magnesium, phosphorus, and other minerals. But doctors can monitor many of these minerals with automated blood tests.

Q   What can patients in hospitals or nursing homes do to ensure that they receive adequate nutrition?

A   Initially, they must communicate their need for adequate nutrition while institutionalized. This involves having meals on time and receiving supplements and between-meal feedings if they can eat only small amounts at the regular mealtime or if additional intake is required. Favorite foods can be brought in by family members, as long as the food conforms to the prescribed diet.

Slurries are an ideal way to include oat-bran and wheat-bran fiber in hospitalized patients' diets. Blend two tablespoons of unprocessed bran or oat bran with a cup of frozen skim milk, then add bananas, blueberries, raspberries, or other fruits. These fruit drinks taste like milkshakes.

Individuals should learn about their nutritional requirements so they will be able to select foods with proper nutritional value from the options available on the hospital menu.

Hospital staff—nursing, dietary, and medical—must view nutrition as an important method in the treatment of disease. Hospital personnel should be nutrition educators, explaining the importance of various foods when serving meals (for example, why brown bread is better than white bread). Hospital units should have refrigerators and microwave ovens available, and whenever possible, encourage families to bring in the patients' favorite foods.

WEIGHT CONTROL

Q   It seems that obesity has become more of a problem in recent years. What has caused this tendency? Also, what is the difference between being "obese" and being "overweight"?

A   Obesity is a condition in which a person's body weight exceeds his or her ideal weight by 20 percent or more. If you are heavier than your ideal weight but less than 20 percent heavier, you are merely "overweight."

Fiber researchers believe more of us today have the tendency toward obesity because we have taken the fiber out of the carbohydrates we consume. Because of this, we eat more calories but we don't feel full. In parts of the world where fiber intake is high, obesity is rare.

Dr. Denis Burkitt, author of *Eat Right to Stay Healthy and Enjoy Life More*, says that the way to avoid obesity is by "leaving the steak and eating the potato." Potatoes are an excellent slimming food. They contain high amounts of lysine, are rich in fiber, and have about as many calories as apples.

Q How can I start losing weight by eating more fiber? My family has a history of heart disease and obesity.

A Starting on a high-fiber, weight-loss diet could be as simple as changing from white to whole-grain bread. Studies have shown that such a minor switch makes a considerable difference in the bulk of food present in the digestive system, even when comparable amounts are ingested. The amount of fiber in the whole-meal bread (four times more than white bread), as well as increased saliva, are the reasons. When bulk in the diet is increased, you are satiated more quickly, thus you will eat less.

Other important additions to the high-fiber slimming plan include bran breakfast cereals, brown rice, fruits, corn, broccoli, carrots, potatoes (especially with their skins), yams, raspberries, and strawberries.

Research at Duke University disclosed the benefits of a rice diet for the cardiovascular system. Eat rice in as many ways as possible, as a reducing food.

CHILDREN AND NUTRITION

Q I have been trying to put more fiber into my family's diet, but our children are picky eaters and have stonewalled my efforts. If two out of four people won't eat a dish, it becomes rather a waste to fix it. How do you add more fiber to a diet that children will eat?

A   A balanced high-fiber diet is important for children as well as adults. A mother from Oregon wrote the following advice to *The Saturday Evening Post:*

Dear Dr. Cory:

I find that plain, toasted wheat bran is a subtle and versatile way to add fiber to my family's diet. Use it generously whenever you prepare hamburgers. Use it to extend and help thicken sloppy joes or soup or meat loaf. It's great when baking too.

Learn to make your own granola. It is very simple and you can put many delightful high-fiber things into it. If your children think they don't like granola, use it as a snack food at first. Chances are high they'll soon change their minds and enjoy it as a breakfast cereal.

Leave the peelings on apples, potatoes, and other vegetables. If [the children] do mind at first, they will probably soon get over it, especially if it is their only option.

Q   My three-year-old daughter is showing some tendencies toward being overweight. How can we help prevent her from being obese?

A   Being obese can lead to a multitude of psychological as well as physical problems. It is particularly impressive that 40 percent of children overweight at age seven and 75 to 80 percent of teen-agers who are overweight become overweight adults. So you are right in trying to catch this problem early with your daughter. Although we know that there are genetic and biological tendencies toward obesity, our environment, behavioral patterns, and food preferences often develop during childhood. Before activity and eating habits are ingrained in a child, he or she should change those that could lead to obesity.

In order to prevent obesity:

- Discourage activities that contribute to excessive caloric intake and decreased energy expenditure, such as eating and watching television at the same time. Not only is watching TV a sedentary activity, but TV advertisements encourage between-meal snacking.
- Do not use food as a reward. Offer nonfood rewards for good behavior.
- Encourage daily physical activity appropriate for the child's age. Involve the child in a regular exercise program, such as playing a team sport, taking a swimming or gymnastics class, or just bicycle riding, jumping rope, or skating.
- Avoid second and third helpings on higher-calorie foods.
- Offer low-calorie, nutritious snacks such as fruit and raw vegetables.
- Try to keep from buying tempting, high-calorie, low-nutrient foods. If they're not around the house, the whole family is less likely to eat them.
- Bake, broil, or steam foods instead of frying them. Use low-fat milk and dairy products. Avoid or limit the use of butter, sugar, margarine, and salad dressing.
- Try to resist offering food when the child is bored or unhappy. Encourage the child to eat only when hungry, and if your child is bored, suggest he or she take a bike ride or play with friends.

Consult your child's doctor who can give you further advice and review her growth pattern. She is in her growing years, so aim for good nutrition and reasonable weight gain for her height.

EXERCISING INFANTS

Q   I exercise regularly and feel that my infant daughter, even at her young age, could also benefit from simple stretching exercises. Could you give me some regular exercises I could do with my daughter?

A   Both you and your infant could benefit from regular mother-baby exercising. It can develop a special bond between the two of you while strengthening your baby's muscles and improving her circulation and coordination.

Here are a few simple exercises taught at YMCA "You and Me, Baby" classes for mothers and babies:

Hug and Rock: Lay baby down and cross her arms in front of her. Holding her arms, gently rock her back and forth. This may calm a crying baby.

Flex and Extend: Hold the baby's ankles and gently bend her knees in toward her chest. Repeat three or four times on each leg at first; gradually increase the number of repetitions. This exercise is good for strengthening thighs.

Legs and Hands: Raise baby's hands over her head, one arm at a time. Lift legs up in similar manner when changing her diaper. This movement may relieve gas and help quiet a colicky baby.

NUTRASWEET™ FOR CHILDREN

Q   Is it safe to give products with NutraSweet to my children?

A   A lot of controversy still surrounds the use of NutraSweet (aspartame). Doctors around the country continue to issue warnings about who should avoid aspartame. The Food and Drug Administration (FDA) maintains that aspartame poses no risks for children, but some FDA officials believe that infants should not be given aspartame. Some consumers of aspartame have complained of a variety of symptoms ranging from headaches and dizziness to nausea and vomiting, rashes, hives, menstrual changes, convulsions, forget-fulness, and depression. They felt their symptoms were related to the consumption of aspartame. Approx-imately 67 percent of the complaints have been neu-rological or behavioral in nature.

The Centers for Disease Control in Atlanta investi-gated more than 500 complaints from aspartame con-sumers and reported that "Although it may be that certain individuals have an unusual sensitivity to the product, these data do not provide evidence for the exis-tence of serious, widespread, adverse health conse-quences attendant to the use of aspartame."

Phenylalanine is one of the two amino acids that make up aspartame. The other is aspartic acid. Consumption of phenylalanine can be a definite danger for children with the inherited disorder phenylketonuria (PKU). Be-cause these children are unable to process foods con-taining phenylalanine, irreversible brain damage may result.

Dr. Keith Connor of the Children's Hospital in Wash-ington, D.C., is conducting studies now on the be-havioral effects of aspartame on children. Preliminary findings indicate there may be some adverse effects. He also "definitely would not advise any pregnant woman to drink aspartame-containing substances" because of the lack of information with regard to the adverse effects of aspartame on a developing fetus.

Until further studies regarding children are completed, it is probably wise to limit children's intake of aspartame, especially if the child experiences adverse effects such as rashes, headaches, hyperactivity, or dizziness.

Products containing aspartame should be stored in a cool place. Beware of any heated products—such as cof-fee or gelatin made with boiling water—containing as-partame because of the sweetener's instability at higher temperatures. Continue to read food labels because an increasing number of products contain aspartame, and unless you read labels, you may consume more aspartame than you realize.

———— C H A P T E R 3 ————

Adult Health Problems

The hope is that new levels of emotional and spiritual maturity go along with increase in age. However, as you reach middle age, aches and pains may begin to occur because of the physical and mental stresses produced by our fast-paced lives and less-than-ideal eating and exercise habits. The following overview of adult health problems is merely a beginning point for gathering information about some of the problems that may arise during adulthood.

PEPTIC ULCERS

Q   How common are peptic ulcers? What are the warning signs?

A   An estimated 4 million Americans suffer from peptic ulcers. About one in ten of us will develop one or more ulcers in our lifetime. Although no one knows why, people tend to get more ulcers in the spring and in the fall.

There are two main types of peptic ulcers. Duodenal ulcers occur within the first few inches of the small intestine. Gastric ulcers occur in the stomach and are most commonly associated with aging. They're rarely seen before age forty and the peak incidence is from fifty-five to sixty-five.

Awakening from sleep with an epigastric (upper middle region of the abdomen) pain is a well-known hallmark of duodenal ulcer disease. Studies have shown that the incidence of both gastric and duodenal ulcers doubled in persons who smoke. There is a correlation between the number of cigarettes smoked and the prevalence of gastric ulcer disease, and we know that it takes smokers with duodenal ulcerations a longer time to heal than nonsmokers. Drinking alcohol or caffeine may worsen the problem of peptic ulcers by stimulating excess acid secretion in the stomach. Studies show that chronic gastric ulcers occur more often in people taking large doses of aspirin.

Treatment used to be linked to large amounts of antacids, bland diets, and surgery. Treatment today is based upon developments of new drug therapies. Tagamet is a very potent inhibitor of acid secretion. Another similarly acting drug is called Zantac. These drugs have reduced the need for surgery, which makes this step forward in medicine especially important.

HEMORRHOIDS

Q Who suffers from hemorrhoids? How do you treat them?

A People who have refined diets, including large quantities of meat, (meat contains zero fiber) commonly suffer from hemorrhoids. Low-fiber diets often result in constipation, and those who are frequently constipated are more susceptible to hemorrhoids. Women commonly suffer hemorrhoids during pregnancy and after labor and delivery. Homosexual males have a far greater incidence of hemorrhoids than do heterosexual males because of their participation in anal intercourse.

Babies are born with their internal hemorrhoids intact. These are a necessary part of our anatomy. They aid in the closure of the G.I. tract much as the lips can form a seal at the beginning of the G.I. tract. These internal hemorrhoids are delicate and can be torn away from their moorings by one's straining on a stool or during anal intercourse. Because internal hemorrhoids occur on mucosa with no nerves, they are usually painless. Often, the first symptoms of these hemorrhoids are bleeding and discharge of mucus.

External hemorrhoids are tan or gray and are easily detectable, small, soft swellings. Thrombosed hemorrhoids result from a blood clot in the hemorrhoid. The clot stretches the sensitive anal skin and causes intense pain, which can appear suddenly.

Hemorrhoids can be treated with sitz baths and topical ointments. To prevent recurring problems, a high-fiber diet resulting in regular bowel habits is extremely important. If these treatments fail, the alternatives aren't pleasant. Surgery to remove hemorrhoids is quite painful as is infrared photocoagulation, rubber-band ligation, and cryosurgery, in which the hemorrhoids are frozen with liquid nitrogen.

Eating bran and whole grain products aids the prevention of hemorrhoids.

GALLSTONES

Q   What type of person has a predisposition to gallstones? What can one do to avoid gallstone surgery?

A   Female, fat, fertile, and forty are the surgeons' four F's of gall bladder disease. Women who have had multiple pregnancies, are overweight, take birth control pills, or have high levels of estrogen are more prone to suffer from gallstones. Dr. Denis Burkitt, a recognized authority on diet and disease, has completed a twenty-year study of the natives of Africa and gives us reason to think that insufficient fiber in our Western diet may be the reason 20 to 35 percent of Americans get gall bladder disease by the age of seventy-five and the African natives do not.

The gall bladder stores bile, which is released in response to eating and aids in the digestion of fats. The most common kind of gallstone is formed from cholesterol in the bile. Some of it is excreted in the bile and a great deal of it is transformed into bile acids.

The body practices a remarkable conservation of bile acids. As they travel the course of the intestines, they are reabsorbed from the bowel and carried back to the liver. The acids are then "recycled" and poured back into the digestive system. The bile acids are re-used several times before they are finally lost in the stool. One of the means of lowering blood cholesterol is to reduce this reabsorption of bile acids. Then as more of the acids are lost through the stool, the liver must have more blood cholesterol to replace the lost acids. As the liver uses up cholesterol at a faster rate, the blood cholesterol level drops.

People with gallstones should avoid fats not only because fats cause gallstones but because they stimulate the gall bladder to contract, which causes the pain of gall bladder colic. Reducing fat intake is a means of avoiding the pain of gallstones.

Increasing the fiber in your diet may do great things for you: It can lower your cholesterol level, thereby reducing your chances of a heart attack, and at the same time, lower your risk of having gallstones, diabetes, diverticulosis, diverticulitis, hemorrhoids, and cancer of the bowel.

"Why risk developing gallstones or any other complications when a diet with the fiber your body needs will usually help prevent the trouble?" asks Dr. Denis Burkitt.

Dr. Burkitt, father of the fiber movement, chuckled when he told us, "The strange thing is when you get gallstones, you are often given a drug called chenodeoxycholic acid. It comes from the bile of oxen in the slaughterhouse. And by taking it, you may get rid of your gallstones." Dr. Burkitt recommends a high-fiber diet, instead, which keeps gallstones from forming. "How much better to provide your own correct bile acids," he said, "than to get a gallstone and then go to the slaughterhouse to try to get rid of the gallstone with the bile from a cow!"

Q   I need to have a gallstone removed, but I don't know what to expect. Is surgery necessary?

A   The good news is that gallstones can be removed without surgery by crushing them with sound-wave lithotripsy equipment. Ask your doctor about gallstone lithotripsy. The high-energy ultrasound shock waves disintegrate the gallstones without damaging the tissue around the stones. If the ultrasound stone crushing can prevent even a small percentage of the half-million gallstone surgeries each year in the United States, it will be a godsend for many sufferers of biliary colic, or gallstone pain. Many young women are inquiring about the gallstone "zapper" because they don't want scars from surgery on their torsos. We like the method because it doesn't require a general anesthetic.

Dr. Tilman Sauerbruch, a gastroenterologist from Munich, whose father and grandfather were esteemed surgeons in Germany, pioneered this new method of gallstone removal. One of the two hospitals in Germany currently doing gallstone lithotripsy bears their family name.

Gallstone lithotripsy is being introduced in eight medical centers in the country. Ask your doctor about the center nearest you, or write the Society for the list of centers.

KIDNEY STONES

Q   How can you prevent the formation of kidney stones?

A   Kidney stones affect up to 5 percent of the U.S. population. Most renal stones have calcium in some form. It is felt that increased urea excretion also plays a role in stone formation. Prevention focuses on keeping the urine dilute, so water intake is essential (in the range of six to eight glasses per day). In some cases, salt restriction and medication may be useful. The decrease of protein in the diet would lessen the amount of urea in the urine, and may also help stop stone formation.

Dr. Barry Brenner, a Harvard kidney specialist, is forging into a new area of preventive kidney care. He believes that we could prolong the useful life of kidneys and postpone the need for dialysis by eating less protein. He points out that there may be a fundamental mismatch between the design characteristics of the human kidney and the functional burden imposed by modern high-protein eating habits. Sustained, rather than intermittent, excesses of protein in the diet cause increases in renal blood flow. This increase requires the reserve capacity of the outer portions of the kidney to be used more or less continuously. He believes that this predisposes even healthy people to a deterioration of renal function.

Urea is the principal waste product the kidneys have to eliminate. The level of protein in the diet determines the amount of this waste. Excessive protein burdens the kidneys with excessive urea.

This problem is often compounded in older individuals who do not drink sufficient water. More water does not make more work for the kidneys; in fact, the opposite is usually true. The water flushes the system and helps the kidneys get rid of waste.

The early warning signs of possible kidney disease include puffiness around the eyes, lower back pain, increased frequency in urination, pain with urination, blood in the urine, and high blood pressure. There are often no symptoms, so your doctor may periodically check your blood or urine to monitor your kidney function. You can easily test your own urine between visits to the doctor to detect protein loss, though this is usually unnecessary. Various types of urine dipsticks are available at drugstores and can be used to monitor urinary protein if you and your physican feel you are at risk.

Q   What new methods are used to eliminate kidney stones?

A   Only a few short years ago the first external shock-wave kidney-stone crushing machine arrived in the United States from Germany. As its name implies, this machine can disintegrate kidney stones without surgery or risk to life. This elaborate equipment targets high-velocity shock waves at the kidney stones, causing them to disintegrate into sand. Patients are able to relax with music while their stones are being eliminated.

This surgery-free, noninvasive technique should not be confused with a method of removing kidney stones called ultrasonic lithotripsy, which involves an invasive procedure that makes a rather large track—about the diameter of a man's thumb—through the body into the kidney to give access to the stone.

Q   Please explain how a dialysis machine replaces the function of the kidneys.

A   Dr. William Kolff, a Dutch physician, invented dialysis, or the artifical kidney. The procedure removes the blood from the body and runs it through filters to remove the impurities and fluids, just as the kidneys would do if they were working properly. Renal shutdown, or kidney failure, causes the urea to accumulate and the potassium level to increase. Because of the urea, the patient will go into a coma, and the high potassium level will interfere with the heart's rhythm, eventually causing it to stop beating. Additionally, the poorly functioning kidney may cause some of the following problems: fluid excess, decreased immunity to disease, bone disease, altered glucose metabolism, anemia, and mental confusion. In short, the entire body system is affected by kidney failure.

At first there weren't enough artificial kidneys (dialysis machines) to keep all of the patients alive. Committees including ministers, physicians, and other community members were set up to decide who should live and who should not. Today, dialysis equipment is available to all, helping to keep persons alive until donor kidneys for transplanting can be found.

Dr. Kolff's latest contribution to society is a dialysis machine that fits like a backpack and enables a person to go about his work or play while being dialyzed.

In the United States, dialysis costs the federal government about $25,000 per year per patient. There are approximately 80,000 people on dialysis, many of whom could come off dialysis if only more transplant kidneys were available.

DIABETES

Q How can persons evaluate their blood glucose levels to determine whether or not they have diabetes?

A Evaluation of a blood sugar in an isolated instance may not lead one to the appropriate diagnosis because the blood glucose fluctuates with eating, stress, and illness. The glucose tolerance test measures glucose levels from a fasting condition (no food or calorie intake for eight to ten hours) with sequential glucose and urine specimens taken at set intervals after a glucose load. Often a fasting specimen and a glucose test two hours after eating are sufficient for diagnosis. A fasting level of more than 140 mg/dl or a nonfasting level more than 200 mg/dl is indicative of impaired glucose metabolism.

Perhaps the single most important development in glucose testing has been the creation of the self-monitoring kits that are now available in drugstores throughout the country. In all systems, blood or urine is placed on a chemically reactive strip or tablet. A color change reflects the amount of glucose present. More and more, experts are recommending blood testing, relegating the less accurate urine tests to those who refuse blood sampling.

Urine glucose testing can provide an estimated blood-sugar level, but it is often misleading and unreliable. Sugar collects in the bladder over a period of time and appears in the urine later, so it does not reflect the blood-sugar level at the moment of urination. Urine testing for ketones is still recommended, however.

There are two types of diabetics: type I, or insulin-dependent diabetics, formerly called juvenile-onset diabetics; and type II, or noninsulin-dependent diabetics, formerly called adult-onset diabetics. Type I diabetes causes the body to produce little to no insulin and to change profoundly because of the extreme glucose overload and acidosis. Type I diabetes usually develops in childhood and is caused by a mixture of genetic and environmental influences. It requires insulin replacement.

Type II diabetes occurs ten times more frequently than type I diabetes and generally develops in persons over forty years old. Type II diabetics have insufficient insulin to properly regulate their glucose balance, but their bodies do continue to make insulin. Oral agents, dietary control, and weight loss are the generally prescribed treatments for type II diabetes, which is largely caused by genetic influences.

Diabetic experts encourage regular exercise, controlled diet, and frequent testing to optimize the insulin or oral agents used for control of blood sugars. There is no definitive evidence that close control of blood sugars will eliminate the many complications of long-standing diabetes. However, it is logical that preventing wide swings in glucose levels would be of benefit to the diabetic and many clinical studies support this. Low blood sugars can be life threatening. The person becomes irritable, hungry, and short-tempered. This may progress to confusion, heavy perspiration, and rapid heart beat. If not recognized and treated with a quickly digested sugar, it can go on to coma, seizures, and possibly death.

Q I've heard that diabetics can become blind. Is there anything I can do to prevent this?

A A recent Gallup poll revealed that the fear of the loss of sight is second only to the fear of cancer. In the United States today diabetes is the leading cause of blindness among adults. Twelve percent of insulin-dependent persons who have had diabetes for 30 years or more are blind.

If you are a diabetic, there are two steps to take to decrease your chances of becoming blind. First, have your eyes checked regularly. An ophthalmologist can detect hemorrhages or scars in the retina, called "cotton patches," which result from bleeding within the eye. Frequent check-ups can reveal abnormal growth of new blood vessels, called neovascularization. If discovered soon enough, blindness can be delayed by burning or cauterizing the tiny vessels with laser therapy.

Cataracts occur more commonly in diabetics and can also be discovered early with regular eye examinations. Diabetic cataracts, or sugar cataracts, differ from senile cataracts in that they form earlier than senile cataracts and result from a sugar glazing of the protein in the lens. The sugar and protein cause a "browning" reaction—like toast browning—but with surgery, the brown-clouded lens can be removed. Maturity-onset, type-II diabetics, as well as juvenile, type-I, diabetics have the potential to suffer from cataracts.

Second, control your diabetes with the proper diet, exercise, and, if prescribed, insulin treatment. Recent studies have shown that maturity-onset diabetes can be controlled, even prevented, by following a diabetes-prevention diet with exercise.

Q   Does a high-fiber diet help to maintain the proper blood-sugar level for the diabetic?

A   Dr. James Anderson of the University of Kentucky leads researchers in the field of dietary fiber for diabetics. He has developed the currently recommended diabetic diet, which calls for 55 to 60 percent carbohydrates and only 25 percent fat or lipids and 10 to 20 percent protein. His diet requires generous amounts of starches and plant fiber and restricts sugar, fat, and cholesterol.

For many diabetics, fat in the diet has been the worst enemy. Fat blocks the action of insulin, so the body cannot burn sugar well after a meal containing a substantial amount of fat.

Dr. Anderson's studies show that most diabetics do better by substituting starch for fat in the diet. The baked potato is fine—minus the butter and sour cream.

Dr. Anderson has also determined that large quantities of fiber slow carbohydrate absorption and reduce serum lipids—thus smoothing out blood-sugar levels.

Although the high-fiber diet is effective for the diabetic, the diabetic should not make any changes in diet without the approval of a physician, particularly if he or she is taking insulin.

HERPES

Q   What is herpes?

A   The herpes virus has been around for thousands of years. The Greeks named it herpes, meaning "to creep." Tiberius Caesar is said to have tried to eliminate it from his land by putting a ban on kissing—manifestly half a measure!

Not all herpes viruses are transmitted sexually. Herpes simplex I causes the familiar, painful fever blister—a topical, recurrent infection that flares unpredictably, generally on the lip. And a third kind of herpes infection is caused by the varicella-zoster variety, which produces chicken pox in children and herpes zoster, the notorious and painful shingles, in adults.

Humans are the only reservoir of genital herpes, or herpes simplex II, infection. The infection is spread through intimate contact, when one sexual partner is having an active outbreak. An active infection is a cluster of painful vesicles or blisters located on the penis, buttocks, anus, vulva, cervix, or vagina. Recurrent lesions are frequent and may involve nothing more than three to twenty days of an uncomfortable, contagious sore. With millions of cases of genital herpes reported in the United States, and the number growing each year, many young people are returning to more conservative social behavior.

Herpes simplex II has several serious effects that have influenced the more conservative attitudes of young people toward the sexual revolution.

For starters, the shedding of the virus through the birth canal of infected women causes fatal or profoundly damaging meningoencephalitis in newborns. When a mother has an outbreak less than two weeks prior to delivery, a Caesarean section is done to protect the baby. Approximately 1,000 babies a year are born with herpes, probably because the mothers were not aware of their infections before delivery. The virus spreads quickly through the infants' systems, killing more than half of them and leaving most of the remainder with permanent brain damage.

Secondly, this organism is thought to cause a fivefold to eightfold increase in cervical cancer in infected women. Doctors recommend that women with herpes get Pap smears twice a year.

Finally, herpes may reveal one partner's infidelity, so the virus can cause emotional strain in a marriage, and even divorce.

Dr. Richard Griffith and his dermatology colleagues

began finding that some people who eat a lot of arginine-rich foods (seeds, nuts and chocolate) need extra lysine to control their Herpes Simplex I.

The physicians scattered throughout the country who now use lysine have reported some positive results. Most of them use 1,500 to 3,000 mg of L-lysine supplement a day (in three doses). To prevent recurrences, they sometimes use as little as 500 mg of lysine per day. In addition, all of the physicians with whom we spoke insisted that decreasing the intake of arginine was equally important in creating a bad environment for the herpes virus.

Dr. Griffith published results of new research on lysine and the prevention of herpes in the October 1987 (Vol. 175) *Dermatologica*.

CHAPTER 4

Surgical Procedures

Most of us will have to undergo at least one type of surgical experience during our lives. Because there is such a cloud of mystery about what happens to us during surgery, we approach the event with trepidation. Much of this fear is unwarranted. Becoming informed about some general surgical practices beforehand will ease the fear and allow us to face the surgery with hope and courage.

DONATING BLOOD FOR MAJOR SURGERY

Q Can I donate my own blood for use in upcoming surgery?

A It may take some effort, but there are good reasons for having your own blood drawn ahead of time to be used for possible transfusion. You can't give yourself an infection that you don't already have, so by donating your own blood for surgery, you eliminate most of the risks entailed in receiving a transfusion. The risks to a blood product transfusion include transfusion reactions, transmission of disease, rare graft-versus-host disease, circulation overload, iron excess, and clotting disturbances (only with multiple transfusion in a short span of time). The first three can be avoided by donating blood to yourself.

Those at high risk for AIDS are asked not to donate blood, but as AIDS spreads to the heterosexual community, more people who do not know they have been infected with the AIDS virus may be donating. Since infected victims may innocently donate blood, we question the safety of the antibody screening tests currently being used to detect the AIDS virus.

We know that after a victim has become infected, there is a period before the antibodies are detectable. This period is called a "window," during which the AIDS virus would not be detected in any tests currently being done on donated blood.

There is another way to receive your own blood during surgery: The surgery staff can collect uncontaminated blood during the surgery and return it to the patient as needed.

AIDS isn't the only reason for recommending autologous blood donations. About 7 to 12 percent of the people receiving blood products contract hepatitis. Because of the blood screening tests, only 10 percent of these infections are hepatitis B. The vast majority of transfusion hepatitis is non-A, non-B hepatitis. As explained by the Centers for Disease Control, it isn't possible to detect non-A, non-B hepatitis in donated blood. No matter how careful the blood banks are, there is no technology at this time to tell which blood is infectious. And it isn't possible to "heat treat" red blood cells to kill this virus because the red cells would be destroyed. Hepatitis B can be prevented by a vaccination if one is deemed at risk. There is no non-A, non-B vaccine.

Red blood cells can be frozen without being harmed, however. If you are contemplating surgery, your frozen red blood cells may be kept almost indefinitely if maintained at temperatures below $-65°C$.

If you expect you'll be needing surgery in the future, it is a good idea to give your doctor plenty of time to arrange for autologous transfusion. Your body's ability to replace lost red blood cells should not be a problem, but if you are anemic, your doctor would likely tell you that you couldn't predonate if your hematocrit level was below 34 percent. Your doctor might choose to prescribe an iron supplement prior to your series of autologous donations so that the chances of your becoming anemic are decreased. Most people replace their red blood cells rapidly after donating blood.

Dr. Douglas Surgenor recently wrote in the *New England Journal of Medicine* about the availability of autologous predonation and transfusion services. He stated:

> The number of currently active hospital-based pre-deposit programs is not known. In 1980, 1 of 10 U.S. hospitals (681 of 6,432) reported collections of autologous blood. It is likely that at least 1,000 hospitals have programs now. The advantages of an autologous pre-deposit program in the patient's own hospital include simplification of the logistics, freedom to make special provisions for patients, and continuous contact between the patient, the blood-bank staff, and the patient's physician. As an alternative, almost all of the 200 regional blood centers in the United States offer an autologous predeposit service to patients by arrangement with the hospitals in their regions.

ANESTHESIA

Q   Please advise me on some of the risks and precautions regarding general anesthesia.

A   Many emergency surgeries come as a result of accidents or unexpected disease complications. Local anesthesia—topical anesthetic or anesthetic injected to numb only the area or region that requires attention—is becoming more popular. But for many surgeries general anesthesia is still the only alternative, particularly when it is imperative to have immobility of the lungs or the heart during surgery.

Some pre-operative precautions include not eating or drinking anything for at least eight hours before surgery. During surgery it would be easy to vomit gastric contents if a person had a full stomach. These gastric contents could be aspirated back into the lungs, creating a lack of oxygen (asphyxia) or a severe type of pneumonia, either of which could lead to death.

Obese persons are at greater anesthesia risk, because more anesthetic is required to keep the muscles in their bodies relaxed. In addition, post-operative recovery is more difficult for obese patients, when movement, coughing, and deep breathing are imperative.

While risks for general anesthesia are slight, there is the reality that one out of ten thousand persons will suffer a cardiac arrest during surgery. Thus sophisticated monitoring devices are used to detect difficulties and intervene when necessary.

A person is monitored to calculate the amount of oxygen being received and to assess the depth of anesthesia. Many other complex tests and evaluations can be done if needed.

In addition to anesthesia drugs, a muscle relaxant is frequently used to make surgery easier for the patient. Sometimes drugs to control blood pressure are used or antibiotics may be administered if necessary.

During the preanesthetic interview, a patient should inform the anesthesiologist of any drugs being taken, both prescription and nonprescription. Some of these drugs can alter the balance of the body and can create problems if the anesthesiologist does not know about them. The patient should also tell the anesthesiologist about any allergies he or she has, about previous surgeries, and if any blood relatives have had undesirable reactions to surgery.

After surgery a patient goes to the recovery room where the staff has emergency monitors. Patients generally stay in recovery for forty-five minutes or longer, until the anesthetic has diminished to a safe level. The patient may then be transferred to a regular hospital room or an intensive care area to continue recuperation. Some surgeries are minor and the patient will go home after he or she is fully awakened, able to move around, able to take fluids, and is reasonably comfortable.

MALIGNANT HYPERTHERMIA

Q   Can a person with a family history of malignant hyperthermia undergo surgery?

A   We have heard of people who don't dare trace their lineage back too far for fear of finding a horse thief in the family. Becoming familiar with the family tree, however, might one day save your life.

If someone in your family history had the rare syndrome called malignant hyperthermia, you too may be susceptible to sudden death in anesthesia if your anesthesiologist doesn't know about your history. This trait has a dominant inheritance pattern; thus if one parent has the syndrome, the child has a 50 percent chance of inheriting malignant hyperthermia. If both parents have it, the offspring's chances rise to nearly 100 percent. The overall incidence of malignant hyperthermia is 1 in 20,000 patients undergoing general anesthesia. Most individuals who have malignant hyperthermia are not aware of it until after being given an anesthetic. Symptoms may not be triggered during the first exposure to anesthesia but may occur at a subsequent one. The symptom complex of malignant hyperthermia is caused by an inherited defect in the muscle and is usually seen when a muscle relaxant is used with an inhaled anesthetic.

In 1983 Ray Naramora was in an automobile accident in Birmingham, Alabama. He needed extensive surgery to repair the cuts on his face and was given a general anesthetic. He had a violent reaction: his temperature shot up to 108 degrees, and he was comatose for five days. The doctors gave him little chance of survival but, miraculously, he did recover. Had Ray known his family history, he would have been aware that his cousin had had a high temperature after getting an anesthetic in 1979. He might have been able to warn the doctors in Alabama about the possibility of malignant hyperthermia.

If someone in your family has had a diagnosed malignant hyperthermia episode, you should consider having the only test believed to show susceptibility to malignant hyperthermia. In this test, a biopsied sample of your skeletal muscle is placed in a bath of caffeine and halothane and stimulated to contract. The muscle response is analyzed, and the diagnosis is usually clearcut. While new centers are being developed, there are at this time only a few that can actually perform this exam. Your doctor can find out where.

People susceptible to malignant hyperthermia *can* have surgery. If the condition is suspected, alternate anesthetic agents can be used. If the syndrome occurs unexpectedly during surgery, the anesthesiologist can take emergency measures, including stopping surgery, cooling the patient with ice, increasing oxygen to the patient, and giving a medicine called dantrolene. Unfortunately, this syndrome can be fatal.

It's extremely important for each person going to surgery to inform his or her personal physician and surgeon of any complications related to rise in body temperature, any complications related to surgery, or the fact that any member of his or her family has had complications.

If you have anyone in your family who's had malignant hyperthermia, it's a good idea to wear a med-alert bracelet to give information to an anesthesiologist who might be suddenly taking care of you following an accident.

PLASTIC AND COSMETIC SURGERY

Q   How do you find a qualified plastic surgeon?

A   Because there are no regulations against it, any M.D. can advertise as a plastic surgeon. Leafing through the yellow pages to find a plastic surgeon can be not only unwise but also dangerous.

In addition to medical school, internship, and three years or more of general surgical training, the board-eligible plastic surgeon trains through a fellowship, lasting two years or more, in plastic and reconstructive surgery. Make sure that the plastic surgeon you consult is board certified or board eligible in plastic and reconstructive surgery. The American Society of Plastic and Reconstructive Surgeons has available a pamphlet on how to select a plastic surgeon.

Consult friends who have already had cosmetic or reconstructive surgery, or you can seek recommendations from your famly doctor. If you're new in the area or do not have anyone to ask, try the local medical society or a nearby large teaching hospital. Patients may also use a referral service operated by the American Society of Plastic and Reconstructive Surgeons. The registry lists members of the society and their specialties. The society will provide you with the names of six surgeons in your area. To make use of the service, either write the society or call its referral service number. The address is: The American Society of Plastic and Reconstructive Surgeons, Patient Referral Service, 233 North Michigan Avenue, Suite 1900, Chicago, Illinois 60601. Their phone number is (800) 635-0635 and is in service twenty-four hours a day.

Once you have chosen a surgeon, you have to make sure that he or she is the right one for you. There is nothing wrong with consulting two or more surgeons to find the one that is best for you. If the surgeon doesn't discuss the advantages and disadvantages of the procedure or starts suggesting a variety of other procedures, you should be wary.

Above all, the experts say, before you consider cosmetic surgery, make sure you have given some thought to the reasons that you want it done. Many insurance companies will not cover a purely cosmetic surgery, so clarify the costs with your surgeon and insurance company early in your decision.

Q   What type of surgeon is required for repair of a facial wound? Can old scars be removed by a competent surgeon?

A   You never know when you may need a plastic surgeon. Accidents are never expected. Any severe facial-wound that is deep, jagged, extensive, animal-inflicted, or dirty should be treated by a plastic surgeon, who has the experience to prevent or to minimize permanent scarring. Injuries involving the eye area may call for a plastic surgeon or ophthalmologist.

If you or a family member suffers a serious facial injury while in a rural area or in a small town where plastic surgeons aren't immediately available, seek medical attention, but realize you may be referred to a different hospital. Stop the bleeding as necessary, but then take time to consult with your doctor or get other help to locate a skilled plastic surgeon, one who is experienced and has the proper equipment to do microvascular suturing if necessary. Take the time to travel; the slight delay will not harm the chances of good repair.

If you've had a facial injury that was hurriedly sutured initially, corrective surgery can still be done years later. Needle holes may be excised and adjacent skin advanced to cover them. Dermabrasion may be used to help get rid of needle holes. Sometimes the original injury is reproduced and restitched. For example, if a lip has been cut all the way through and sutured badly, a plastic surgeon will simply take it all apart and put the vermilion line, the muscle, and the skin back together aesthetically. Corrective surgery of this nature should be done no sooner than six months after the original injury so that the tissue has had time to regain its soft, pliable nature.

ORGAN TRANSPLANTS

Q   I believe that giving your kidneys, heart, or lungs when you no longer need them could be giving the gift of life to someone. How do you feel about this?

A   You are so right! Giving your kidneys or your heart or your lungs when you no longer need them could be giving the gift of life.

The bright new star in the field of organ transplantation is a new drug, cyclosporin. It opposes the body's rejection of a donated organ, permits healing to take place, and allows normal resistance to infection.

The greatly improved success rates with organ transplants have swelled the demand for organs far beyond the supply. When kidney transplants were first tried, only 50 percent functioned after one year. At that time the kidney had to come from a near relative. Now four out of five kidney transplants from all donor types are functioning a year after their implantation. Fortunately, people who don't have a kidney can be kept alive for several years on dialysis machines, thus allowing time for a suitable organ to be found.

France, Italy, Israel, Poland, Norway, and Austria have enacted "presumed consent" laws. These allow organs from the bodies of accident victims to be donated unless the victims' families have documents forbidding the use of the organs.

Today forty countries have joined a network to share information and to exchange organs so that each recipient gets the organ most likely to be successful, and each organ is placed where it is least apt to fail and be wasted. It is not uncommon for a donor kidney from California to be implanted in a recipient in Florida or Pennsylvania. The Walter Reed Army Hospital uses a military jet aircraft to pick up and transport donor organs to any location in the United States where a matching recipient is waiting.

The need for organ donations is sure to grow as the success rates of transplantation improve. The problem belongs to everyone, as we are all potential recipients in need of an organ.

I've signed the donor permit on the back of my driver's license and so has my husband. However, when an accident occurred, neither my husband nor I thought about an organ donation. When one of my husband's kidneys was removed, he could not have thought of donating it because he was unconscious. I should have thought to donate the kidney, but I was too emotionally involved. That healthy kidney went to the path lab, when it could have gone to a person who needed it badly. What can we do to avoid such oversights from happening? What policy could be instituted to prevent such an unconscious error? Perhaps we should have a presumed consent law as practiced in some of the European countries.

Q   Under what conditions can a person have a lung transplant? How successful is this type of surgery?

A   Poorly functioning lungs and oxygen starvation can be caused by asthma, emphysema, cystic fibrosis, and primary pulmonary hypertension. Of all the reasons for severely impaired lung function, the most common one is emphysema.

Today there are thousands of emphysema patients needing new lungs who should be watching the work of Dr. Joel Cooper with great interest. He persevered doing lung transplants on animals and bravely pursued the transplantation of lungs in humans at a time when many transplant surgeons were too discouraged to try. (Heart-lung transplants are not as difficult.) Recently he has successfully performed double-lung transplants on emphysema patients. His work has been done at Toronto General Hospital. He will move soon to St. Louis.

MICROVASCULAR SURGERY

Q   What are the chances that a limb can be reattached to the body after being severed in an accident?

A   Annually, thousands of home and industrial accidents result in the loss of a person's life or limb. For those whose limbs are severed, there is now hope of replantation and return of function.

Fifteen years ago, emergency room personnel might have been sadly amused that a victim of an accident would even bring in a severed finger, toe, or hand, hoping to have it sewed back in place. Standard procedure was to dispose of the severed member and close the stump as quickly as possible.

Today, thanks to new developments in microvascular surgery—careful mending done under a large microscope with microscopic needles and thread—severed members can often be restored with return of function.

Microvascular replantation centers have been established across the United States. You are rarely more than two hours away from a center. A list of their locations could well be the most important item in your first-aid kit. For major accidental amputations, jet ambulance planes, fully equipped with intensive-care units, are available.

Immediately wrap the severed limb in a moist sponge or cloth, preferably sterile. The limb should then be placed in a plastic bag and the bag immersed in ice water. Do not close the bag off as the part should have oxygen. The part should not be allowed to freeze or soak in water. After stabilization from the injury, the patient with his amputated part should be brought at once to the nearest hospital where arrangements can be made for transportation to the nearest center for microvascular surgery.

Haste is important, but if the severed part is kept cool (close to 39° F) it can be replanted up to twenty hours following the accident.

The following points are important to remember:

1. Place the severed part into a damp cloth or sponge.
2. Then put this into a plastic bag or any other water-proof container.
3. Place the open container in a pail of ice water.
4. The part must have oxygen. *Do not close the container.*
5. Do not let the part freeze: Ideally it should be kept at 39° F.
6. Never soak a severed part in water.

CHAPTER 5

Women's Health

A woman's body is physiologically more complex than a man's body and can have more complications relating to the reproductive system than a man's. The following questions and answers reflect some of the physical problems women experience.

YEAST INFECTIONS

Q Several of my friends have contracted yeast infections, but I'm embarrassed to admit I don't know what a yeast infection is. Can you explain?

A You may be most familiar with the word yeast in connection with baking bread or the fermentation process to produce alcohol. You may be surprised to learn that this microscopic relative of the vegetable kingdom lives in our bodies. In most of us, the yeast cause no problem; they're controlled by friendly bowel bacteria. But since the widespread use of birth control pills and antibiotics that destroy bacteria, troublesome yeast infections have become common.

Previously, diabetics and pregnant women were most likely to have these infections. Now yeast infections occur in teen-agers who have been taking an antibiotic such as tetracycline for their acne and especially in women who have been on birth control pills. A common yeast infection is vaginitis. A yeast infection can also occur in the colon, where it causes gas, bloating, and alternating diarrhea and constipation. The fermentation of the yeast causes bloating, and victims may notice their belts becoming too tight. The yeast most often causing problems is called *Candida albicans,* a Latin term for "glowing white." This yeast occurs even in healthy people and can be found in the throat, mouth, gums, fat folds, nose, vagina, gastrointestinal tract, and other mucous linings. The yeast does not cause problems until something happens to the body's immune system or natural colon bacterial balance.

Steps taken to cure chronic yeast infections generally include going off the pill and avoiding antibiotics whenever possible.

BIRTH CONTROL

Q   What are some methods of birth control other than the pill?

A   AIDS has created a resurgence of demand for barrier methods of contraception, particularly condoms. The combination of condoms and spermicidal gel or foam and the diaphragm makes a highly effective birth control technique. Contraceptive devices linked with intercourse are more prone to failure because of user compliance. Rhythm and withdrawal methods are not recommended for couples who would not accept a surprise pregnancy. Abstinence, though not a popular means of birth control, remains the most effective means of preventing pregnancy.

A new method of birth control presently being investigated at a number of medical centers in the United States involves plugging the Fallopian tubes with a small amount of liquid silicone. The silicone gels to block the passage of eggs from the ovaries down the tubes into the uterus. It is done as an outpatient technique and requires no general anesthesia or invasive surgery.

The procedure itself is performed by the physician who places a small amount of local anesthetic in the cervix to prevent pain. Then the doctor inserts a lighted instrument known as a hysteroscope through the vagina and cervix into the uterus. Through this hysteroscope, the doctor passes a small plastic tube into the uterine opening of the Fallopian tube. A small amount of silicone is then allowed to flow through the plastic tube and into the Fallopian tube. The silicone solidifies in several minutes, and tubal blockage is thus accomplished. A special loop is imbedded within the silicone to allow for later removal.

Silicone has been used in the human body in various ways, for a number of years. A nontoxic substance, silicone doesn't cause local tissue reaction nor does it adhere to the surrounding tissues.

The silicone plug may be inserted in a physician's office, and the entire procedure usually takes no more than forty minutes. No recovery period is necessary before resuming normal activities.

PAINFUL BREASTS

Q   I am in my twenties and I have very sharp pains going through my breasts. I told my doctors about it, but they said not to worry. I asked for x-rays and they refused. What can I do?

A   Do you drink a lot of caffeinated beverages? Fibrocystic change is a benign, noncancerous condition that is a frequent cause of breast pain. Sometimes painful fibrocystic change can be eliminated or improved by simply removing all caffeine from the diet. Some women have found relief from painful lumps in their breasts by taking 600 units of vitamin E per day and eliminating all caffeine.

Breast discomfort that occurs during the premenstrual time is a natural body response to that portion of your menstrual cycle. Although it may seem inconsequential, wearing a poorly fitted bra will cause discomfort, so be sure to invest in a good support bra.

Lastly, if you feel the doctors did not adequately address your concern, either return to your physician or see another physician who will listen to your complaints and explain his or her diagnosis to you. Any physician will change his or her advice over time if a symptom persists, so please return for further explanation, examination, and therapy: ultrasound, mammography, or biopsy might be considered appropriate. Occasionally, doctors will prescribe medical therapy with birth control pills or other hormones if the other above methods do not successfully provide relief.

Q   What precautions should I take against breast cancer? I'm fifty-five years old.

A   I hope soon to see the mammogram become as popular as the Pap smear, which has saved thousands of women in the past twenty years from death because of cervical cancer. The next time that you're with a large audience of women, consider the fact that one out of every ten will get breast cancer. If you are a female over fifty years of age and you aren't having a yearly mammogram, you're playing a kind of Russian roulette. The older we get, the greater our chance is of having breast cancer: women in their eighties are at a much greater risk of breast cancer than women in their thirties, for example.

The National Cancer Institute is studying the effects of diet on women who are very high risks for breast cancer. Half of the very high-risk participants are trying to achieve 20 percent fat diets to see if that will reduce their cancer rates.

Because all women are in a high-risk group, they should maintain a low-fat/high-fiber diet and be careful of the amount of caffeine they consume. Women should give themselves a monthly breast examination, and if they find a lump, they should go to their doctor immediately.

ENDOMETRIOSIS

Q   After I tried for several years to conceive a child, my doctor began to suspect that I might have endometriosis. What can you tell me about this problem?

A   Endometriosis is sometimes called the executive woman's disease because as many American women postpone marriage and pregnancy to launch their careers, they increase their risk for endometriosis and fertility difficulties.

Endometriosis is a puzzling disease that is most prevalent in women between thirty and forty years of age but that can occur in the teens and twenties.

It is believed that during monthly periods small fragments of the uterine lining are pushed out of the uterus back through the Fallopian tubes. These fragments then implant on the tubes, on the ovaries, and in the abdominal cavity. The tissue continues to respond to the hormonal changes of the menstrual cycle. Over time, areas around the implants become inflamed and scarred. Women who have endometriosis have a 50 percent infertility rate.

Laser laparoscopy is a relatively new technique that enhances fertility in women with endometriosis. For diagnosis, a laparoscopy, a tube with a light in it, is inserted through a small incision in the umbilicus. If endometriosis is discovered, a laser is used to vaporize the endometrial implants and scarred tissue. This is an outpatient procedure, and there is less chance of adhesions forming than when open abdominal surgery is performed in a laparotomy. Surgical gynecologist Dr. Leo Bonaventura explained: "You use an incision through the belly button that may be only about a centimeter or less in length. You put a second incision, if you use double puncture, just above the pubic bone that's about half a centimeter. You put the laser through the one, the laparoscope through the other. And then you direct the laser at the tissue that you're trying to vaporize."

When asked about the indications for laparoscopy in diagnosing endometriosis, Dr. Bonaventura responded, "Women will go to their local physician and he'll say 'O.K., we think you have endometriosis.' Well, thinking is not good enough. You cannot diagnose it by an exam—it has to be by laparoscopy. The symptoms are pain, irregular periods, painful intercourse. Those are probably the three most common; of course, infertility is definitely suspect. If they have any of those symptoms they should be seen."

Until a few years ago, a total hysterectomy was the only treatment for severe endometriosis. Now, however, a hysterectomy is the last resort. Hysterectomies are relegated to those individuals who have so much disease that it involves the bowel and bladder. Endometriosis can cause damage to these and other organs.

BREAST FEEDING

Q   I've heard that breast milk is superior to formula because it contains nutrients that formula does not. What are the differences between breast milk and formula?

A   Mother's milk is the perfect food for newborns. Although formulas have been greatly improved over the years, they still do not contain all of the factors present in human milk. One factor missing in formula is lactoferrin, a whey protein that promotes the absorption of iron and inhibits the growth of harmful bacteria in the intestines. Formulas have zinc added, but the infant does not absorb it optimally because of the absence of the zinc-binding factor that is present in human milk. Breast milk also has the right level of copper, so important for premature babies. Breast milk can also help prevent anemia. Even infants up to six months old that are fed an iron-fortified formula may develop iron-deficiency anemia because the baby is less efficient in absorbing iron without the presence of the lactoferrin in breast milk.

The protein content of human milk is low (about 6 percent) but is of high nutritional quality. The low protein and high water content make breast milk easily metabolized and managed by young kidneys. Many minerals in breast milk are present in lower quantities than in cow's milk but are better adapted to the babies' needs.

Cow's milk has little iron available, and it appears to decrease the absorption of iron from other foods. Whole cow's milk should not be given to an infant before six months of age because the milk is too high in protein and does not have enough carbohydrates. Casein, a protein in cow's milk, forms a large curd in the stomach that's hard to digest.

About 15 percent of children may be *sensitive* to cow's milk, but children often outgrow this. Less than 5 percent of children are actually *allergic* to cow's milk. They have such symptoms as recurrent vomiting or diarrhea, eczema, and recurrent colds, colic, bronchitis, or asthma. A cow's milk sensitivity may also show up in the child if the breast-feeding mother drinks cow's milk. Approximately one-third of breastfed infants with colic may be reacting to cow's milk consumption by the mother. The culprit seems to be whey protein, the most sensitizing of cow's milk proteins. Although allergies are hereditary, studies show that allergy-prone children do much better at resisting allergies when given breast milk.

One of the most important advantages of breast feeding is the resistance to infection that it builds in the young child. Colostrum, the clear protein-rich fluid that precedes the milk, contains many of the mother's antibodies that it passes on to the newborn. Breast feeding within the first hour after birth increases resistance to infection and helps to avert the decrease in blood sugar, which frequently occurs soon after delivery. The mother's antibodies in the milk continue to work for the baby until he is developed enough to produce his own. Anti-infection factors in breast milk protect against such viruses as polio and herpes and several bacterial infections.

We also tend to overfeed bottle babies. Babies who are breast fed naturally set the pace for feedings and weight gain. Interestingly, breast milk composition changes from feeding to feeding, as well as during the feeding. The higher protein milk comes first, and the more satisfying, higher fat milk comes at the end of the nursing.

Breast feeding is good for the mother, too, because suckling stimulates the release of oxytocin, which in turn causes the mother's uterus to contract. These contractions help to control bleeding after birth and firm up her stretched muscles.

La Leche League International has done much to encourage the return of breast feeding by informing mothers of the physical advantages of human milk as well as of the important relationship between mother and baby that breast feeding establishes. Princess Grace of Monaco bought the La Leche League manual when she was expecting her first child. After breast feeding all of her children, she was a strong supporter of La Leche League. Her speech at their international convention in 1971 did much to popularize breast feeding and make it acceptable to modern women.

LOW BIRTHWEIGHT

Q   My first child was small at birth; he weighed only five pounds. Is there anything I can do during pregnancy to ensure that my next baby won't be underweight?

A   Expectant mothers can take the following steps to reduce the chance that they will have an underweight infant:

1. Stop smoking cigarettes. Many experts believe the incidence of low-birthweight infants could be reduced by 25 percent if pregnant women did not smoke.
2. Practice good nutritional habits. Expectant mothers who eat properly and gain weight appropriately during pregnancy are far less likely to give birth to an underweight infant.
3. Prenatal care should begin as soon as a woman knows she is pregnant. Experts increasingly recommend that couples who are planning a family should consult their family physician or an obstetrician before trying to conceive.
4. Abstain from alcohol. About 5 percent of low-weight births are linked to alcohol consumption during pregnancy.
5. Avoid any medication or drug (nonprescription, prescription, or illicit) unless under the specific direction of an obstetrician.

Seven out of every one hundred infants born in the United States are underweight at birth. Many factors, both maternal and fetal, can cause low birthweight. Infants who weigh less than 5.5 pounds at birth have a substantially greater risk of suffering from a number of medical problems.

ESTROGEN THERAPY

Q   As I approach my late forties, I want to know more about the use of estrogen as a "helper" through the menopausal years. What considerations and benefits should I weigh in my decision about whether to take estrogen?

A   Might estrogen prevent memory loss? Might it even prevent Alzheimer's disease and heart attacks? Dr. Howard Fillit, who is a geriatrician—an internist specializing in the problems of old age—spoke on the new indications that estrogen skin patches might be used for many menopausal and postmenopausal women. We were so impressed with his work I'd like to share it with you.

When he finished speaking, one woman in the audience said, "I'd put on a skin patch tomorrow if I thought it would help me remember my shopping list." It has been discovered that women with a severe memory loss due to Alzheimer's disease have lower estrogen levels than those who have escaped this dreadful affliction.

Dr. Fillit explained that getting estrogen into the system can now be accomplished in a manner far better than in past years—by using a transdermal skin patch that makes use of the skin as a gateway to the body. Many physicians believe this skin patch, just approved by the FDA, will revolutionize the way menopause is treated. It delivers estrogen through the skin directly into the bloodstream, simulating the way ovaries deliver estrogen to the blood. Although the patch has a very small amount of estrogen, it effectively eliminates or reduces such symptoms as hot flashes, night sweats, and vaginal dryness. It is about the size of a silver dollar and is worn on the abdomen and changed twice a week.

We asked Dr. Fillit about the side effects of estrogen:

With the patch, the drug enters directly into the bloodstream; therefore, a woman avoids many of the side effects associated with her taking the drug by mouth. What happens when women take estrogen by mouth is that the estrogen goes from the stomach into the liver. In the liver 90 percent of the estrogen is converted from the naturally occurring form into a metabolite that probably has little if any estrogenic effect and may have its own side effects. . . . When the estrogen goes into the liver, it induces the liver to synthesize many different proteins involved in abnormal clotting and perhaps in hypertension and some of the gall-bladder problems that can be associated with routine estrogen therapy by mouth.

Dr. Fillit also commented on how many postmenopausal women he believes should be on estrogen: "Probably most of the women should be on estrogen-replacement therapy," he said. "I believe the new data show estrogen-replacement therapy is safe and effective and may prevent many of the complications of long-term estrogen deficiency, such as osteoporosis."

Before estrogen-replacement therapy, women must have a thorough physical exam along with a mammogram. As with all medications, estrogen-replacement therapy may not be appropriate for all women, especially women with a history of certain cancers. If you're taking estrogen and want to change to the skin patch, talk to your doctor. The patches are now available by prescription.

OSTEOPOROSIS

Q   I have read several articles alerting women to their need for calcium and of the possibility of their developing osteoporosis. I'm not sure if my diet has adequately provided the calcium I've needed over the past several years, and my grandmother had a dowager's hump. How can I find out if this disease has already begun in me?

A   Have you ever wondered what doctors will do when cures are discovered for cancer, emphysema, diabetes, and heart disease? In such a case, the new screening device developed to test women for osteoporosis should keep thousands of physicians busy.

Osteoporosis, involving a loss of calcium from the bones, afflicts one out of every four white women who reach the age of sixty. It is rarely diagnosed in black women.

An x-ray won't reveal osteoporosis until more than one third to one half of the bone has disappeared. Fortunately, instruments called densitometers can detect as little as 1 to 2 percent of bone loss. The individual's arm is placed between a sealed radioactive source and a gamma ray detector. Although the technique relies on radiation, the exposure is only about .01 percent of the exposure of a conventional x-ray. The procedure takes five to ten minutes and is completely painless.

An immediate print-out indicates whether bone mass is normal, low, or intermediate. Repeated measurements of the same areas will permit calculation of the annual rate of bone loss.

Since osteoporosis is preventable but not curable, early diagnosis is vital. Screening should start at about age thirty-five and be repeated every two or three years until the onset of menopause. For the next two years, tests should be done every three or four months. Once the rate of bone deterioration has been determined, a yearly densitometer evaluation is recommended.

If you're a postmenopausal white woman, you should be tested yearly. Black women have little problem with osteoporosis because their initial bone density is greater than that of white women and the loss that occurs with aging is less significant.

INFERTILITY

Q   What are the causes of infertility? I have been trying to get pregnant for seven months, but to no avail. My husband and I are tired of our friends saying, "Just relax!" What should we do?

A   For approximately 3½ million American couples, or about one out of every five couples, the joy of being expectant parents is lost to feelings of personal inadequacy, guilt, and even resentment toward one's spouse when experiencing infertility for months or even years. However, thanks to recent medical developments, infertility does not have to rob many of these couples of one of marriage's richest rewards.

An estimated 40 percent of infertility cases are strictly male-related. Yet in many of the remaining couples, subtle problems in each reproductive system may amount to a major problem inhibiting a successful conception.

The apparently healthy couple who has had unprotected intercourse three times weekly for twelve months or more without conception may consider themselves infertile and should seek the help of a recognized fertility specialist. These doctors are ably prepared to diagnose and prescribe treatment for many kinds of infertility.

Keeping a basal temperature chart (for women) is one of the first steps in solving fertility problems. By recording daily her morning temperature, a woman's actual time of ovulation, and thus her maximum time of fertility, can be determined. This simple task done faithfully can produce the right timing for sexual relations and may be all that is lacking to allow the long-awaited conception. Your gynecologist or infertility specialist will find this information extremely useful.

Some of the conditions leading to female infertility are endometriosis—a condition wherein aberrant uterine tissue spreads from the uterus to block the Fallopian tubes—and such pelvic inflammatory diseases (PIDs) as gonorrhea or chlamydia, which may cause scarring and permanent closing of the tubes. Gonorrhea and chlamydia both respond well to drug therapy, as long as treatment begins early.

Microvascular surgery can, in some cases, be used to

repair or restore Fallopian tubes that have been scarred or blocked by PID, endometriosis, or tubal ligation.

In several institutions around the world, doctors are able to help couples who cannot conceive because of irreversibly blocked Fallopian tubes. An egg can be removed from the woman's ovary, fertilized by the man's sperm outside the body, and then deposited into the woman's uterus. This process of in vitro fertilization bypasses the need for a patent (open) Fallopian tube.

For many infertile women, the problem is an imbalance between reproductive hormones to create normal, timely ovulation. In these cases Clomid, a synthetic hormone, is used to trigger the ovulatory cycle and then may be followed with the use of Pergonal, which matures the egg in its follicle and readies it to drop through the Fallopian tube for insemination.

In the male partner infertile conditions may include a varicocele, a varicose vein in the scrotal sac that allows warm abdominal blood to collect. The slight elevation in temperature actually destroys the available sperm. Surgical correction of the varicocele can restore fertility. In addition, men who wear briefs that are too tight may be overheating the sperm in the testes by pulling them too near the body's core heat, thus inhibiting normal seminal production. The testes should maintain a temperature that is lower than the body's core temperature for optimal sperm production.

Quite frequently a blocked vas deferens, the tube through which semen passes from the testes to the urethra, will inhibit insemination. Again untreated gonorrhea or chlamydia may be the cause of such blockage.

And finally, faulty semen can cause infertility. Misshapen and weakly active spermatozoa cannot reach a fertile egg and impregnate it. Recent treatment with Clomid and Pergonal for the male has produced good results in restoring a vital, healthy seminal fluid.

ECTOPIC PREGNANCY

Q   What are the dangers of an ectopic pregnancy? Under what conditions is one most likely to develop this condition?

A   When a fertilized egg begins to grow in the Fallopian tube, the embryo can rupture the tube so that blood rushes into the abdominal cavity. The result may be fatal if surgery is not quickly performed.

Several years ago I had a house guest who developed a pain in her lower back and above her rectum. I thought, "ectopic pregnancy," but at first ruled it out because she insisted that she had just had a menstrual period. She wanted to fly out of town the following morning, but I was fearful for her to leave without a pregnancy test.

A pregnancy test quickly revealed—to her great surprise—that she was pregnant. Unfortunately, the fertilized egg had implanted on her ovary and ruptured, causing bleeding into the abdominal cavity. Had she boarded the plane, she could have died from internal bleeding. She had emergency surgery and has since had children without further difficulty.

The most common ectopic pregnancy occurs when the fertilized egg becomes attached to the walls of the narrow Fallopian tubes that lead to the uterus. The embryo may even attach itself to the ovary, the broad ligament, the intestines, or the cervix. The egg may become joined to the inside of a normal tube or where the tube is rough and scarred from an infection. If the egg is fertilized, it begins forming a baby. As the baby grows, the tube stretches to the point of rupturing and bleeding begins.

Because of blood loss, the woman generally goes into shock, necessitating an immediate trip to the nearest hospital for emergency life-saving surgery.

The frequency of ectopic pregnancies has increased

threefold over the past fourteen years. There are now about fifteen such pregnancies for every one thousand live births. One reason for the increase may be the intra-uterine contraceptive device (IUD). Although these devices prevent uterine pregnancies by keeping the lining of the uterus agitated so that the fertilized egg cannot find a nesting place, they do not prevent the egg from attaching itself to the Fallopian tubes. Further, the increase in the number of abortions and sexually transmitted infections caused in large part by multiple sexual partners and changing moral values have contributed to the rising incidence of ectopic pregnancies.

CAESAREAN SECTION

Q What are the reasons for so many C-section deliveries?

A Many ask why it is necessary for 20 percent of the babies born in the United States to enter in this "unnatural" way.

If a disproportionate relationship, called CPD (cephalopelvic disproportion), exists between the fetal skull and the mother's pelvis, a safe vaginal passage is not possible. Attempting to have the uterus force a large baby through a normal birth canal or a normal sized baby through a too small passage may cause injury to the baby and may subject the mother to an unnecessarily long, painful labor. Pelvic bones misshapen by injuries or by a disease may make birth canals impassable for the baby.

A woman in labor is monitored closely on several parameters. The baby's position is carefully assessed, and the mother's vital signs (blood pressure, temperature, and pulse) are monitored regularly. Alterations in the pattern or progression of labor may require rapid surgical intervention to protect the mother and baby. The fetal heart tracing is watched to determine the baby's reaction to or intolerance of the labor process. Changes in this tracing may indicate the need for altering the labor, again in the best interest of the soon-to-be-born child.

Some babies begin their journey through the birth canal in odd postures. Ideally, the baby proceeds down the birth canal with the back of the head (called the occiput) coming first, preferably with the occiput to the front of the mother's pelvis. This is the most favorable position for easy passage through the birth canal.

If the arm or the shoulder present first, the baby comes to lie crosswise in the pelvis and vaginal delivery is impossible. Left to nature, both mother and baby will die.

Babies coming chin first or brow first have considerable hazards as do babies born breech or buttock first. A breech baby has the risk of having the cord fall out and become compressed, thus shutting off the baby's oxygen supply. The baby's legs and hips usually deliver easily, but delivering the shoulders with the arms wedged up beside the head is extremely difficult. Sometimes the head itself is too large to be born after the rest of the baby has been delivered. These problems lead doctors to favor Caesarean sections for babies in these positions at the beginning of labor.

Medical considerations also prompt obstetricians to surgically deliver babies. For unknown reasons, some babies of diabetic mothers die in the womb as the time for delivery approaches. Caesarean delivery a few days early may avoid this complication. Similarly, babies of RH-sensitized mothers and mothers with toxemia do better if delivered before term.

A mother with a vaginal herpes infection that flares up within two weeks before the expected time of delivery is advised to have a Caesarean section to prevent the baby from contracting the herpes. Disseminated herpes can be fatal for newborn infants.

Following a Caesarean section, most doctors prefer to deliver subsequent babies by Caesarean section also.

However, recent studies have shown that perhaps as many as 80 percent of women who have had C-sections could safely deliver subsequent babies vaginally. This partially depends on the type of uterine (not skin) incision, since one to two percent of mothers delivering vaginally after having had a Caesarean suffer torn uteri from the scar left by the former delivery. This is a grave hazard for mother and baby. A woman who has had a Caesarean section can have a safe vaginal delivery, but she and the obstetrician must be motivated to work closely together for a successful delivery.

Childhood Diseases and Related Problems

Infants and children are plagued by numerous illnesses and physical problems that can usually be cured when an informed parent not only offers comfort and love but also takes the responsibility to treat the problem or seek professional medical advice. The following information offers some basic guidance for some of the common diseases and problems beginning in earliest childhood.

FEVERS

Q   Is there a difference between baby aspirin and regular aspirin for a baby's fever?

A   The only difference between baby aspirin and adult aspirin is the number of milligrams of aspirin in each tablet and the vehicle of product. Baby aspirins are designed to be chewed, so they crush easily and have a pleasant taste.

A new government-sponsored study indicates that children given aspirin for chicken pox and influenza face a significantly greater chance of contracting Reye's Syndrome—a serious, sometimes fatal disease—than those who do not receive aspirin.

Albert A. Pruitt, M.D., chairman of the American Academy of Pediatrics Committee on Drugs and the chairman of the Department of Pediatrics at the Medical College of Georgia, said, "The study strongly indicates that aspirin can no longer be regarded as an appropriate medication for children or young adults with flu or with an illness which might be chicken pox. Because aspirin is largely self-medicated by young adults, it is important that the labeling read by the consumer be unambiguous on this point."

Q Should a child with a fever be sponged with water or alcohol?

A A child should never be sponged with rubbing alcohol. The child might inhale or absorb enough fumes to cause a coma a serious reaction.

A common error in treating a fever is to sponge with cold water which causes shivering because the body thinks it is cold. The shivering then raises the body temperature. Always sponge with plain, tepid water. If a child begins to shiver as he or she is sponged, the water temperature should be raised, or the sponging stopped and a cool washcloth placed over the forehead instead.

APPENDICITIS

Q Is there anything a person can do to prevent appendicitis in children?

A Fiber can lower appendicitis risk in children. A new study by researcher Jean Brender of the Audie Murphy VA Hospital in San Antonio shows that children ages seven to eighteen who eat a high-fiber diet have a 30 percent lower risk of appendicitis. Brender and his associates studied the diets of 135 young people with appendicitis and 212 with no appendicitis. They found that those who ate a diet very low in cereal grains and other high-fiber foods had almost twice the risk of appendicitis.

Fiber appears to lower appendicitis risk by hastening the transit time through the intestine of waste products, thus decreasing pressure upon the appendix, the researchers pointed out in the *American Journal of Public Health*.

CHICKEN POX

Q   What causes chicken pox?

A   Chicken pox, or varicella, is caused by a highly contagious herpes virus. Chicken pox is considered contagious the day before the rash breaks out until all the blisters have scabbed over—usually about seven to ten days. If exposed to someone with chicken pox, you will probably contract the disease within 12 to 21 days.

In general, children have less severe symptoms than adults. Children usually get an initial fever from 101° to 103° F and develop a blistery, itchy rash. To prevent infection and scars, do not allow your child to scratch; trim his or her fingernails and bathe the child daily. Applying lotion or taking antihistamines may soothe the itching.

As noted in the section on fevers, do not give your child aspirin products during this illness.

Infection with chicken pox creates lifelong immunity to that form of varicella. Scientists are currently testing a varicella vaccine that may be released for general use in the near future.

CROUP

Q   What is croup?

A   Croup is a generic word for several types of relatively acute infections characterized by a "croupy" (barking) cough, which may be accompanied by hoarseness, harsh respirations, and signs of respiratory distress.

A disease of the temperate zone, croup occurs most often in winter, and more frequently in boys. When people refer to "croup" they are usually talking about acute laryngotracheobronchitis, found most often in children between the ages of five months and five years, and acute spasmodic laryngitis, found most often in

93

children between the ages of one and three years. Both are primarily caused by viruses.

Most people with acute laryngotracheobronchitis have coldlike symptoms for several days prior to the onset of the barky cough, harsh respirations, or respiratory distress. The child can become very restless and frightened as the infection progresses. His or her fever may range from 100° to 104° F. The symptoms are worse at night and often recur with decreasing intensity for two or three nights. Family members may also have coldlike symptoms.

Acute spasmodic laryngitis can cause someone to have a similar cough but a different presentation and disease course. Cold symptoms in the child and the family usually are not present. An easily excitable child seems more prone to this type of croup. There also seems to be a family predisposition to this syndrome. It usually occurs with a sudden onset in the evening or night. The child awakens with the characteristic barky, brassy cough and noisy, labored breathing, and he seems frightened and anxious. There is typically no fever. The symptoms gradually diminish within several hours. The following day he may seem fine except for a slight cough and hoarseness. Similar, less powerful attacks may occur over the next two nights. It is not unusual for such episodes to recur several times.

Most children with acute spasmodic croup or with mild laryngotracheobronchitis can be treated at home. Steam from a hot shower or bath in a closed bathroom, hot steam from a vaporizer, "cold mist" from a nebulizer, or the cold night air usually relieves the child's distress within minutes. The return of such episodes may be attenuated or prevented by one's placing a vaporizer near the child's bed. If the steam or cool night air is not successful, the child's doctor should be called, and the child should be taken to the emergency room.

EAR INFECTIONS

Q   Our grandson has had a chronic problem with ear infections. His doctor does not think he needs tubes in his ears, but we wish something could be done to treat his pain. Do you have any suggestions?

A   Putting tubes in a child's ears is one of the most common operations performed in the country today, says Dr. Richard Miyamoto of Indiana University. However, because of the vastly improved antibiotics available for treating ear infections, most doctors now initially attempt a conservative, nonsurgical approach. The antibiotic the doctor prescribes should relieve the pain in a short time. Until the antibiotic brings relief, analgesics such as acetaminophen may help. Sometimes pain-relieving ear drops can be prescribed. It is important to give your child the entire amount of the antibiotic prescribed to optimally treat the infection.

The issue of a child's receiving ear tubes may be viewed from several perspectives. A youngster with recurring episodes of otitis (or ear infections) who responds well to antibiotics, the infection clearing completely between episodes, rarely needs tubes. A child whose medicine alleviates the infection but whose middle ear continues to collect fluid must be watched carefully for several weeks after the infection. If fluid is retained for two to three months, then surgical drainage and tube placement (after a hearing assessment) may be necessary. If an ear infection won't go away after several different courses of treatment, then the youngster may need surgical drainage and tube placement.

Tube placement is a surgical procedure in which small polyethylene or metal tubes are placed in the ear drum to allow air to get in to the middle ear space. This helps to keep the lining of the middle ear dry and less prone to infections. Although the use of ear tubes has become commonplace, there are still risks involved. A conservative approach is usually best as most ear problems diminish with age.

Q How do you prevent swimmer's ear?

A After swimming, try to get all of the water out of the ear canals by turning the head to the side and pulling the lower earlobe in different directions to help the water run out. Dry the opening to the ear canal carefully. Avoid using earplugs when swimming, because they tend to jam earwax back into the canal. An ear drop can safely be used to prevent swimmer's ear. Use one-half isopropyl alcohol and one-half white vinegar. Two to three drops should be placed in each ear after swimming or showering. A hair dryer may also be *carefully* used to dry the ear canal.

MUMPS

Q What causes mumps?

A A contagious disease, mumps is caused by a virus present in the saliva and the secretions of the nose and spread by direct contact with a person who has the disease. Mumps, commonly occurring in the winter and spring, causes a painful swelling of the salivary glands, usually the parotid glands, located just below and in front of the ears. Fever, muscle pain in the neck, headache, and an overall feeling of malaise are the first signs of the disease.

As with other children's diseases, mumps is a much more serious disease for adults than for children. Males, for example, are prone to suffer orchitis (testicular swelling), which can lead to male fertility problems, if they contract mumps after puberty. Babies are temporarily protected from the disease through their mother's immunity. At fifteen months of age, a child can be given a safe vaccine in the combined MMR vaccine (measles, mumps, rubella) to protect against mumps. Once a person contracts mumps or is vaccinated, the immunity is life-long.

STREP THROAT/TONSILS

Q   How can I keep my child from getting strep throat?

A   Streptococcal pharyngitis (strep throat) is a bacterial throat infection spread by respiratory contact and requires close contact with another person who has an active case of the disease. Strep throat may also be called tonsillitis, a term applied to other types of throat inflammations causing sore throats and fevers. Approximately 15 to 30 percent of the throat infections may be a bacterial (strep) throat; the remainder are caused by viruses. Keeping your child away from persons with sore throats and any objects those persons have handled, particularly objects that have been in their mouths or near their faces, will help to prevent your child from catching their infections.

Q   Why are doctors not performing tonsillectomies as frequently as they used to?

A   Doctors' attitudes concerning tonsillectomies (the surgical removal of the tonsils) have changed dramatically during the last three decades. The once commonplace surgery is today much more rarely performed. Still, there are some children who doctors believe should have their tonsils removed. Deciding who falls into that group, however, is a subject of considerable controversy.

Tonsils are not purposeless blobs of tissue as doctors once thought; rather, they are lymph nodes that act as filters, preventing bacteria that may collect in the throat from gaining access to the bloodstream. Thus the current trend is to treat these infections with medication rather than with surgery. The trend away from tonsillectomies was also prompted by a recognition of the risks associated with surgery and anesthesia and, most important, the uncertainty of the benefits of the procedure.

Tonsillectomies might be advised for children with unusual complications, such as having tonsils so large that they block the airway. But doctors most commonly recommend tonsillectomy for individuals who experience frequent and severe infections because tonsillectomy is an attempt to decrease the incidence of strep throat.

Doctors at the University of Pittsburgh examined the effects of tonsillectomies versus antibiotic medical therapy in children with frequent severe tonsillitis (seven episodes in one year or three per year in each of the preceding three years). They found that tonsillectomies reduced the incidence of strep throats in these children in subsequent years. Children treated with antibiotics instead of surgery also had fewer throat infections, but not as significant a decrease as the tonsillectomy group. The doctors emphasized that only a small number of children have as many throat infections as the group they studied. Furthermore, the doctors did not advise what should be done for the children with fewer sore throats, a subject they are currently researching.

It is important to realize the difference between viral sore throats and strep throats. Tonsillectomy doesn't seem to help the child with frequent viral infections.

Q   I received a notice in the mail that I should bring my children in for HIB vaccinations. Do you think this is a good idea?

A   Yes. The Centers for Disease Control in Atlanta and the American Academy of Pediatrics recommend that all children ages two to five receive the new Hemophilus influenza type-B (HIB) vaccine. Hemophilus influenza type-B (or H flu) bacteria causes more than half the cases of meningitis in young children, as well as other serious complications such as bone, joint, and skin infections; pneumonia; and epiglottis, a severe lower throat infection. The vaccine, though similar in name to the flu shot, is not the flu shot. It aids in the prevention of a group of severe bacterial infections as listed above.

CIRCUMCISION

Q   My husband and I are expecting a son this summer, and we are getting a lot of pressure from my family to have our son circumcised. They say his chances for infection are much greater and that other boys will make fun of him if he is not circumcised.

My husband is not circumcised. His father was a doctor who thought circumcision was unnecessary. I really don't want to circumcise my son, but I'm concerned that my relatives might be right. Any advice?

A   Since the late 1970s both the American Academy of Pediatrics (AAP) and the American College of Obstetricians and Gynecologists (ACOG) have stated that circumcision neither improves health nor prevents disease, and that routine circumcision is no longer medically justified. Circumcision is on the decline among infants in the United States. However, the United States is the only country where a majority of male newborns are still being circumcised for nonmedical and nonreligious reasons.

The practice of circumcision became popular after World War II for "health and hygiene" reasons. In fact, circumcised newborns may be at greater risk for skin infection than uncircumcised newborns, according to a study conducted by six pediatricians who examined

1,343 hospital-born infants at the Tripler Army Medical Center in Hawaii. Their findings, published in the October 1985 issue of the *Hawaii Medical Journal*, indicate that hospital circumcision may be "the culprit responsible for the increased rate of staphylococcal infection of newborn males," a rate of infection that is more than double that of female babies or uncircumcised male babies. Other rare complications of this procedure include hemorrhage or structural damage that often results in the need for corrective surgery later in life.

Based on the fact that there is no medical reason for circumcision, there are a growing number of insurance companies, such as Blue Shield of Pennsylvania and the Prudential Insurance Company, that will no longer provide reimbursement for the cost of routine, nonreligious circumcision.

Contrary to popular belief, the uncircumcised penis needs very little special care. Regular bathing is all that is required for good hygiene. However, parents should never force back the foreskin of an infant or a young child. This can cause tightness and may make circumcision mandatory. (Circumcision after the newborn period normally requires general anesthesia, which carries a whole new set of risks.) The foreskin of the penis will gradually become retractable on its own as the child matures. Complete retraction usually occurs by adolescence.

Uncircumcised babies sometimes experience temporary redness and irritation of the penis, but this is usually insignificant and goes away without treatment. If it persists, it may be a sign of infection, for which your physician may prescribe an antibiotic or a simple bathing.

As for your concern about the child's self-image when around circumcised males, you don't need to worry. Studies on this subject conclude that being uncircumcised does not contribute to a poor self-image.

Circumcision is a personal choice. Although traditions change slowly, now that there is a change in the financial support of circumcision, we may be seeing fewer infants subjected to this painful procedure.

PINWORMS

Q   Lately my little boy has been waking up in the middle of the night crying and itching at his rectal area. Can you tell what this might mean?

A   Your son could be showing symptoms of pinworms.

Pinworms, medically termed enterobius vermicularis, are estimated to infect 5 to 15 percent of the American population, but precise figures are lacking. Other reports claim as high as a 50 percent infection rate in school-age children. Contrary to the popular belief that pinworms affect only dirty and poor people, the worm is found in all social and economic classes.

The pinworm is a thin, yellowish white worm, one-half inch long. A pregnant worm may carry as many as 17,000 eggs. Some of the mature worms, which inhabit the appendix and the large intestine, work their way out of the rectum to lay their eggs on the perianal skin. The eggs rarely survive more than two days in humid conditions and are the cause of the scratching. They are transmitted through ingestion or inhalation from clothing, bed linens, or contact with an infected person's hands. The most common way the infection is spread is for the child to scratch his rectal area, get the eggs on his hands, and then touch something others might put in their mouths.

A symptom of infection includes nocturnal rectal itching that may even awaken the person. Since the worms are large enough to be seen, the infection is diagnosed by actually looking for them at the child's anus. The worms come out onto the skin at night to lay their eggs so the best time to check the child is late at night, after the child is asleep, or early in the morning hours, before the child is awake.

If no worms are seen three nights in row, a simple test can be done by dabbing the sticky side of a 2.5-inch strip of transparent (not translucent) Scotch tape onto the rectal opening. This procedure should be done before the child gets out of bed in the morning and certainly before bathing. The tape can then be affixed to a clear microscope slide, and a lab technician can look for the eggs on the slide with the microscope. The slide needs to be hand-delivered to the lab that very day. If it is mailed, there is a possibility the eggs might hatch en route.

Once the diagnosis is made, by seeing either the worms or the eggs, the condition can be treated by one of several prescription medications. Many physicians will treat not only the clinically infected person but also the entire family.

Besides drug therapy, good handwashing is important. Cut your child's nails short so eggs cannot thrive or lodge under the nails. You can kill eggs on clothes and linens by washing in 132° F water for a few seconds (boiling water is 212° F). Vacuuming or damp mopping of carpets is important because the ova can get into the carpet.

RINGWORM DISEASE

Q   I am a preschool teacher needing information about ringworm disease.

A   Ringworm is a treatable fungal infection marked by the presence of one or more dry, mildly red, and sometimes elevated scaly patches that form a ring around a central clearing—thus, the name ringworm. Children are more susceptible to this disease before the onset of puberty. Ringworm appears on the face, trunk, or upper extremities.

Ringworm can also affect the scalp, where it needs

special treatment. Ringworm of the scalp usually affects children, is contagious, and may become epidemic. Hairs become brittle and break off, leaving broken stumps of lusterless hair. If not treated, large sores may develop on the scalp, causing permanent hair loss. Ringworm of the body is often transmitted by cats or dogs. Ringworm of the feet is commonly called athlete's foot.

Drugs can be prescribed to treat ringworm.

BABY POWDER DANGER

Q I overheard a doctor saying that the use of baby powder should be abandoned. Why?

A The danger is that the talc, if inhaled, can irritate the baby's airway. Dr. Cotton, in a recent letter to the *New England Journal of Medicine*, pointed out that baby powder is especially dangerous for the rare infant who goes home with a tracheotomy because the tube provides a direct, unprotected line to the lungs. He cited the death of a baby from just such an incident. The risk for an infant with a normal airway is much smaller, but the fine grained powder, if inhaled, can irritate the child's lower respiratory tract causing a cough or wheeze.

Although baby powder is widely used for babies in diapers to absorb moisture and keep the skin lubricated and odor free, the actual effect is minimal and short-lived. Because it is not a necessary infant-care item, it is definitely not worth the risk of harm to a baby. If it is used, always put the powder on one's hand and then smooth it onto the youngster's skin; never shake the powder directly onto the child.

TEETHING

Q At what age do infants begin teething? I've heard conflicting information on this issue.

A   Primary or "baby" teeth may begin to erupt as early as three months of age. But most children begin teething between six and twelve months of age. The age at which teeth begin to grow in is usually a family trait. If a child begins teething after this period, it would be a good idea to have him checked by his doctor to discern any nutritional or metabolic disorders.

Parents often believe a drooling child is a teething child. This is not always true. Salivary glands and muscle reflexes that initiate swallowing and lip closure mature when the child is between three and six months of age. At that time, the flow of saliva is increased as a response to discomfort, nausea, or irritative lesions in the mouth. However, excessive salivation will also occur with teething.

Q   My pediatrician advised me not to use teething gels. Can you tell me why?

A   Many of the teething medications contain the local anesthetic benzocaine. Although the risk of poisoning is quite low, teething medicines containing this drug are potentially harmful, particularly since the dosage is not measured. A six month old was reported to have been poisoned like this already. Many doctors are beginning to demand that adequate warning be placed on teething products. But other less controversial comfort measures can be used.

Q   Can teething cause a fever?

A   There is no scientific basis for this commonly held belief. Fever is a useful defense mechanism that alerts us when our body is responding to the onset of a disease, not to a naturally occurring process. Fever is defined as a temperature more than 100.4° F rectally or 99.6° F orally. Lower temperatures, often called fevers, are normal body fluctuations.

THUMB SUCKING

Q   My daughter is eighteen months old and sucks her thumb. At what point should I encourage her to stop?

A   Thumb sucking satisfies an infant's oral desire, which is primary and natural at this age. A child usually sucks his or her thumb while holding on to a "lovey" or a blanket. But as the child matures, the habit usually dissipates, so the parents should not worry. Thumb sucking that continues beyond the age of two, however, is often related to a child's feeling bored or anxious— perhaps the parents' being overprotective or overdemanding—or is done at times when the child wants to feel secure, such as bedtime or when his surroundings are changing.

Up to the age of four, thumb sucking is not usually considered harmful to the teeth or jaw structure. However, older children's thumb sucking may require minor orthodontia.

Because your daughter is still very young, scolding or physically restraining her will confuse her; she has no idea that you would be concerned about her thumb sucking. Assure yourself she is satisfying a need. If she continues to suck her thumb as she grows older, however, note the pattern of her thumb sucking (bedtime, boredom, new situations). She may have some unrecognized insecurity that would require your attention.

Q   Do you have any suggestions for thumb suckers? My three-year-old daughter seems to suck her thumb regularly during the day. My husband and I are worried about orthodontic problems. I've heard that the bad-tasting medicines don't work. Is this true?

A   Thumb sucking is a normal, usually temporary, habit of early childhood. It may be a sign of being tired, bored, thirsty, hungry, anxious, or jealous of a sibling. The child may need more time alone with parents or more time for play with other children. Studies have suggested that medicine that coats the thumb should not be used on children under the age of four, except in the rare case when orthodontic problems are evident. If the habit continues beyond the age of four, most pediatricians recommend considering treatment in order to prevent orthodontic problems such as an overbite.

The adversive treatment involves painting the thumb (or finger) nail with a bad tasting polish, available at your local drugstore. Explaining to your child what you are doing and why is critical. Paint the nail several times a day, and compliment your child when she does not suck her thumb: small rewards or treats are acceptable. You can also remove your child's fingers or thumb from her mouth after she is asleep. But don't nag her or constantly pull her thumb from her mouth and remind her to stop when she is awake. Constant negative feedback interrupting a coping or comfort mechanism can hurt a child's self-esteem. Relapses occur so be prepared to treat the problem again.

SLEEP PROBLEMS

Q   I have a healthy eight month old who continues to wake up at night. He was sleeping through the night well by six weeks. After having had a bad cold and cough he seems to be in this habit of waking up and is not satisfied until my husband or I give him a bottle. Any suggestions?

A   A healthy eight month old who is gaining weight well does not need a night feeding. It sounds as though your child developed a "learned pattern" after being comforted when waking at night during his illness. An infant who relies on being rocked or given a bottle in order to fall asleep will also require them when he has brief wakings (as most adults also do) during the night.

Your baby needs to learn how to fall asleep *in his own bed*. Rocking or nursing your child or giving him a bottle or pacifier at bedtime is fine, but he should be put in his bed (without a bottle) when he gets drowsy. That way he will learn to rely on his own resources to fall asleep. Being put to bed with a favorite blanket or stuffed animal can also gradually help the child "separate" more easily at naptime or bedtime. He may cry after being placed in his bed, but only periodic, brief reassurances are needed from you until he learns to fall asleep on his own. Allow him to cry for progressively longer periods between the times you check on him—five minutes the first night, ten minutes the next, and so on. Do not remove him from the bed or feed him. Offer a few comforting words, a pat or a stroke; then leave. Please avoid any food or liquid other than a few sips of water from a cup.

Because consistency is very important in getting fast results with this behavioral change, the same routine should be followed for all nighttime wakings. A consistent bedtime ritual as well as a quiet time prior to bedtime is also helpful. Night lights are useful. Some medicine or some medical problems such as chronic middle ear disease are disruptive to sleep, so check with your doctor if any of these conditions apply to your child.

Q My two year old has difficulty sleeping at night. How common is this in children her age?

A Most childhood sleep problems are harmless and short-lived. But when sleep problems persist for months, parents should evaluate their child's daytime activities. Daytime stress can cause children, as well as adults, to have trouble sleeping.

According to recent studies, sleep problems seem to occur more often in children who have experienced one or more of the following specific situations: psychological withdrawal of the mother; an accident or illness affecting a family member; an unaccustomed absence of the mother during the day, such as a mother's returning to work or to school; a parent who is frequently depressed; and their sleeping with their parents.

Sleep problems that last a month or longer might indicate that the child is encountering too many stressful situations. In such a case, perhaps the best advice for the parents of the troubled sleeper is to discuss the problem with their pediatrician. Shorter-lived problems are probably best handled with patience and consistency. Try to avoid prolonged attention to your little one when she awakens. You don't want your well-intentioned comfort measures to imply that you are happy with being up at 2:00 A.M.!

BED WETTING

Q   My eight year old has a bed wetting problem. What can I do?

A   Bed wetting, or enuresis, is a common problem occurring in 30 percent of children at age 4, 10 percent at age 6, 3 percent at age 12, and 1 percent at age 18. Boys experience this condition more than girls do, and often one of the parents of a bed wetter was also a bed wetter as a child. It is more common for children to never achieve nighttime control than to be dry for months or years and then begin having difficulty again. The following discussion relates to those who have never achieved control.

Most children who are bed wetters have small or immature bladders and a tendency to sleep deeply. Their bladders won't hold much urine, and the signal to urinate does not come through strong enough to rouse them. Because these youngsters have never had a prolonged period of dry nights and rare conditions sometimes are the cause, parents and children need to consult with their physician about the problem.

There are many ways of dealing with this condition, including motivational counseling, bladder exercises, medications, and nighttime alarms. Current trends favor alarms and motivational counseling. But your doctor will be able to determine which treatment will work best for you.

Most children gradually stop bed wetting as they grow older, so you shouldn't worry excessively. Meanwhile, restrict your child's intake of caffeine, which is found in chocolate and in many soft drinks, because it acts like a diuretic and stimulates urination. It is advisable for your child to avoid overexhaustion before bedtime and for you to take him to the bathroom just before he goes to bed.

You might want to use a large towel lined with plastic to eliminate the need for the frequent changing of the entire bed. Although your child does not intentionally wet the bed, most experts encourage children to take responsibility for their habit by changing and laundering their sheets or by helping to do this, depending on their age. You should keep a calendar record and star and compliment the dry nights, downplaying the accident nights.

CONSTIPATION

Q   I'm the mother of two healthy children. They are both good eaters, but my five year old seems to have recurrent problems with constipation. Any suggestions?

A   Constipation often occurs because of a lack of fiber in your diet and/or a sudden decrease in the amount of exercise you get, as happens when you become ill, for example.

By eating more bran, whole grain, fresh vegetables,

and fruits, the amount of your dietary fiber will increase. The fiber adds bulk to stools, which makes them easier to pass on a regular basis. Drinking fluids such as juice and water is also helpful.

Wheat bran or corn is very high in fiber, so it makes a wonderful natural laxative. It can be found in, or used with, many foods, such as cereals, muffins, oatmeal, casseroles, brown rice, or whole-wheat bread. Some good fresh fruits and vegetables to help fight constipation include prunes, figs, dates, raisins, peaches, pears, apricots, beans, carrots, lettuce, spinach, and cabbage.

NOSEBLEEDS

Q   My youngest child, age three, gets occasional nosebleeds after roughhousing with his older brother. What is the best way to stop a nosebleed in a young child?

A   To start, blow all of the blood out of the nose. Then, pinch the tip of the nose so that both of the nostrils are closed. Keep the nose pinched for ten minutes to allow a plug clot to form in the broken vessel. If bleeding resumes, blow out all the blood and pinch the nose again for ten minutes. Afterward don't blow the nose or pick it, or the clot may be torn off and the bleeding resume.

Your child should be sitting up with his head tilted slightly forward when you are trying to stop his nosebleed. This creates less pressure in the nose and keeps blood from draining down the throat.

If these methods do not work, you should contact your doctor, who may try to pack the nose with adrenaline. The packing puts pressure on the blood vessels in the nose and slows down the blood flow. The adrenaline causes the bleeding arteries to contract, and stops the blood flow, hastening the formation of plug blood clots to seal the ends of the ruptured vessels.

Ice packs on the back of the neck are unnecessary, but you can place a cold cloth on the nose and pinch "over" it for ten minutes, as mentioned above. After a nosebleed, gently apply vaseline inside the nostril to help reduce recurrences.

PINKEYE

Q   How long is a child with pinkeye contagious?

A   A child with pinkeye, or conjunctivitis, is usually not contagious after twenty-four hours of treatment with an eye medication or after matter has stopped forming. However, prior to that time the discharge from the eye is highly contagious. The infected child should have separate bathroom towels and bed linens. He should be encouraged not to touch or rub his eyes, and he should wash his hands often, to prevent the spread of infection.

COLORBLINDNESS

Q   Upon entering kindergarten this year, my five year old was discovered to be colorblind. Could you give me information on this problem?

A   Colorblindness is an X-linked genetic defect, meaning that it is passed on by the mother's genes. Of the mothers that carry this gene, approximately half of their sons will be colorblind and half of their daughters will carry the gene but not have the disorder. The defect occurs in 8 percent of white males and in only 0.5 to 1 percent of white females. Colorblindness is usually partial, with problems occurring most frequently in red-green discrimination.

Teachers are usually first to discover colorblindness in children. There is no treatment, but parents, teachers, peers, and relatives should know that the child's perception of color is different from that of others. The individual's lack of proper perception of traffic lights and car brake lights may be of particular concern to family and friends. In no way should colorblindness be considered a form of developmental or academic failure, but rather a comparatively minor handicap.

BIRTHMARKS

Q My three month old was born with pinkish birthmarks on his eyelids and the back of his neck. My pediatrician said they were fine, but I wonder if they will always be there and if they will get bigger?

A Fifty percent of newborns have these salmon patch markings, known as "angel kisses" when on the eyelids and "stork bites" when on the back of the neck. These marks also appear on the face, between the eyebrows, just above the nose. When the infant cries they become more noticeable because of increased blood flow to the skin, but they do not enlarge. Most eyelid patches fade within the first year of life. The patches above the nose and on the back may persist longer and may reappear transiently when bloodflow to the face increases. No therapy is needed.

HEAD LICE

Q What do you recommend for treating head lice?

A Head lice, or *pediculosis capitis*, commonly infest the hair of children and often are difficult to eradicate. Part of the difficulty comes from the continued prevalence of head lice in the community, but the other part of the problem is due to incomplete treatment of the affected child. The two main agents that have been available for treatment are effective but may require several applications in order to completely eradicate the parasite in all stages of its development. The nits, or eggs, hatch within seven to ten days into mature nymphs that go through several molting stages before maturing into adults in about two weeks. Soon after becoming adults, the lice mate, and within a day, the females begin to lay eggs. One female may lay up to 150 eggs during her one-month life span. It is important that the medication be not only pediculicidal (killing the lice) but also ovicidal (killing the eggs). That way the life cycle can be stopped and the parasite eradicated.

In addition to prescription medications, several over-the-counter preparations with varying costs and effectiveness are available. Contact your physician for recommendations.

Some schools require that all of the nits be removed from the hair before a child returns to school. There is a possibility with some medications that the nits could hatch and that reinfestation could occur.

The other important part of lice treatment is cleansing the environment. Lice can live up to forty-eight hours away from the host, and nits can live up to seven days away from the scalp at room temperature. All washable clothing and bed linens should be machine washed in hot water or dried for at least ten minutes in a hot dryer. The nonwashable items should be kept in airtight bags for ten days or dry cleaned. Combs and brushes should be soaked and washed in a pediculicide. Carpets, upholstery, and mattresses should be vacuumed thoroughly.

Some physicians recommend treating only the child's roommate or anyone else with a visible infection, whereas many physicians recommend treating the entire family.

BEE STING

Q What should I do if my toddler is stung by a wasp or a bee?

A   The greatest number of these stings happens in August. Severe reactions are more likely to occur in persons over thirty years of age.

If your child is stung, watch to see whether or not he has an anaphylactic reaction (exaggerated or severe response to a foreign protein, such as histamine). These reactions are most likely to result from yellow jacket stings, but also result from bee, wasp, and hornet stings. This reaction rarely occurs after a bite from other insects. Call your physician and take your child to the nearest emergency room immediately if he has been stung more than five times by the insect or if he shows any of the following symptoms of an anaphylactic reaction:

- difficult breathing
- wheezing
- tightness in the chest or throat
- hives, swelling, or itching *elsewhere* on the body, away from the site of the sting
- weakness, feelings of anxiety, abdominal cramping, or loss of consciousness
- previous serious allergic reaction to this insect

Anaphylactic symptoms are generally present within fifteen to sixty minutes of the sting. If the stinger is still present, remove it before you take your child to the emergency room. Do not squeeze the stinger with tweezers because more venom could be squeezed into the bite, but scrape it off with your fingernail instead. Once the stinger is removed, apply an ice cube to the site to slow the absorption of the venom. If you have any antihistamines or cold medication with antihistamines, give one dose immediately. If you have an anaphylactic survival kit, use it as previously instructed by your physician.

Even if a reaction is less severe than an anaphylactic one, it is still important to remove the stinger (often seen as a black dot in the center of the bite). After removing the stinger, rub the area for fifteen minutes with a cotton ball soaked in a meat tenderizer to relieve the pain. Ammonia or ice rubbed on the area also brings relief. If your child remains uncomfortable because of persistent itching, use aspirin (in this case aspirin acts as an anti-inflammatory agent, which acetaminophen would not do) in combination with an antihistamine.

Continue to watch your child for symptoms, as some studies have reported an onset of severe reactions up to twenty-four hours after a sting. Local reactions consist of a sharp pain, localized swelling (bites on loose tissue such as the eyelid can cause pronounced redness and swelling), and redness with later hardening of the tissue around the bite. Wasp, hornet, and yellow jacket stings are frequently infected by bacteria, so continue to monitor the bite for infection. A tetanus booster may be necessary as well, so check with your doctor even after a minor bite.

To help prevent bites from these insects:

- Wear shoes while out-of-doors.
- Avoid gardens, orchards, and garbage.
- Avoid scented soaps, lotions, perfumes, or cosmetics.
- Avoid brightly colored, loosely fitting clothing.
- Keep car windows closed.
- Have an exterminator destroy hornet or wasp nests in and around the home.
- Keep a survival kit available, particularly if the child is known to be sensitive to insect stings.
- A child who is sensitive to stings should wear a Medic-Alert bracelet or necklace that records the insect allergy.

PLANTAR WARTS

Q   What are plantar warts? How can you get rid of them?

A   Warts are growths on the surface of the skin caused by a virus. They are spread by person-to-person touching or sometimes by touching an object with the virus on it. Plantar warts grow on the soles of the feet and are often quite painful. More than 50 percent of warts will disappear on their own within two years. However, an untreated wart may spread to other areas of the body.

If you have a plantar wart, contact your doctor who can prescribe a topical therapy combined with soaking and scraping. Occasionally the physician may "freeze" the wart. Cutting the warts out or trying to remove them vigorously is usually not recommended because permanent scar tissue can result.

Treatment does not guarantee that the wart will not return. But despite the occasional discomfort, these warts are not dangerous.

SEXUALITY

Q   My five year old is beginning to ask questions about sexuality. Do you have any advice for how I should handle this subject?

A   It is normal for your child to be asking questions about sexuality at this age. Likewise it is common for parents to feel unsure or awkward about how to respond. Don't let these feelings shut off this important communication. This is a marvelous opportunity for parents to share beyond the issues of anatomy and function by providing accurate, loving information about our natural feelings. Sexual responsibility and morality are indeed best taught at home, with reinforcement at school and/or church.

Try to keep these points in mind when discussing sexuality with your child:

• Don't be afraid to admit that you don't know everything.

- If you're embarrassed, say so—your child will sense it anyway—but then go on to address his questions.
- Begin by being aware of what your child already knows—his concerns, interests, and level of understanding. Resist the temptation of quizzing him, however.
- Tell your child what he wants to know—no more and no less.
- Let your child know that it is O.K. to discuss sexuality with you.
- Use accurate terminology for body parts and functions, even when your child is young.
- Don't use animals as examples to illustrate human reproduction. (Animals should be used to explain animal reproduction.)
- Children don't always initially ask what they really want to know, but the initial discussion doesn't need to include everything. There will be many opportunities for further discussions.
- Discuss the private and public aspects of sex talk and behavior.
- If your child asks questions at an inappropriate time, be sure to set a definite time for your discussion and then stick to it.
- Give information before your child experiences various stages of puberty (such as the first nocturnal emission or menstrual cycle). Books can be very helpful in conveying information or stimulating discussions. Your librarian should be able to recommend several.
- Give moral guidelines for sexual behavior. Children feel more comfortable knowing why sexual activities are to be delayed and that their parents support certain lifestyles.
- Give information about both sexes to your child. It is natural for children to be interested in what's happening to the opposite sex, as well as to their own.

Eyes, Ears, and Teeth

This chapter focuses on the care of three important areas of our bodies: the eyes, the ears, and the mouth. Through these orifices we experience some of the most pleasant sensations life has to offer. And with the proper care, we will extend the longevity of these body parts to experience the bounties of this world for many years.

Q   I have never had any problems with my vision, but my wife insists that I visit an ophthalmologist to have my eyes tested. Is this necessary?

A   If eyes are the windows to the soul, they are also windows to what's going on in your body. The people who boast that they haven't seen a doctor for ten or twenty years often are missing good opportunities to prevent serious conditions in their later years, including blindness or a premature death.

The eye is the only place in the body where, without surgery, arterial blood can be seen flowing through naked blood vessels. With an ophthalmoscope, a physician can peer inside your eye, look at the small vessels, and possibly detect disease early. Through the eyes, the doctor can actually see hardening of the arteries. This condition can cause the vein beneath the small artery to be compressed. Doctors refer to this as "nicking."

In a normal state, the vessels of the eye are clearly defined and unbroken. Cholesterol forming in the arteries or high blood pressure can cause the artery walls to harden and thicken. A low-fat/high-fiber diet can lower serum cholesterol levels and prevent hardening of the arteries.

As discussed in chapter 2, under "Diabetes," the retina of the diabetic's eye reveals scars called "cotton patches," which are a result of bleeding within the eye. Ophthalmologists can also detect in the early stages abnormal growth of new blood vessels, called neovascularization. Burning or cauterizing the tiny vessels with laser therapy can delay blindness.

Even after you have had your eyes tested and the results show 20/20 vision, you may still have eye problems. Early glaucoma can affect the occurrence of tunnel vision, in which you will have 20/20 vision in the center of your visual field but be blind at the periphery. People with glaucoma sometimes experience blurred and foggy vision, and occasionally the glaucoma victim will see halos or rainbow-colored rings around lights.

Glaucoma occurs when the body has too much fluid inside the eye. Pressure begins to build and eventually destroys the eyesight. In order to measure this intraocular pressure, the doctor can use a tonometer and anesthetize the eye before the measurement, or the physician can use an airblast tonometer, which measures the pressure painlessly, without an anesthetic. Glaucoma occurs most frequently in adults over thirty-five who have a family history of glaucoma. A glaucoma test should be a part of your annual physical exam.

Some doctors have observed that people who work in the sun for long periods develop cataracts on the lower portion of the lens where the eye has been exposed to direct sunlight. If you work or play in the sun a lot, you can have an optometrist coat your glasses with a clear, nondetectable coating, developed by NASA, that filters out harmful ultraviolet light.

If you have cataract surgery, in which the eye's lens is removed, you will need UV protection or your retinas will absorb unwanted UV radiation. Because the pupils are damaged in cataract surgery, they can no longer constrict in bright light.

The following symptoms require an eye examination by an ophthalmologist:

- pain in or around the eye
- sensitivity to light
- light flashes
- blurred vision
- continual redness
- floaters (little black dots that float across the visual field)
- excessive tearing

If you have photophobia or light-sensitive eyes from taking medication, if your spouse reads while you want to sleep, or if you travel at night on airlines, a pair of shades is helpful.

Q   My three month old seems to have trouble focusing her eyes on objects. Is she too young for me to be concerned?

A   Even newborns and infants are susceptible to eye problems such as crossed eyes or squint (strabismus) and lazy eye (amblyopia). The earlier these conditions are treated, the better.

During the first few months of life, when a child is learning to use both eyes together, it's normal for the eyes to appear crossed or out of alignment from time to time for brief intervals. If by three and a half months the misalignment appears frequently, is long lasting, or is always with the same eye, the infant should be examined by an ophthalmologist.

Lazy eye is the lay term for the condition causing children to have crossed eyes or one eye that is more nearsighted or farsighted than the other. It can be diagnosed in the newborn, or it may develop later in a person's life. Lazy eye can be treated with special corrective prisms, contact lenses, and exercises. The stronger eye is often covered with a patch to stimulate use and strengthening of the wandering eye. Some parents have found that it helps a young child to adjust to the patch if they wear one themselves.

Any time you are concerned about the way your child's eyes move or focus, visit your doctor.

CONTACT LENSES

Q   Are there advantages to extended-wear lenses as compared to the regular soft lenses? Are contact lenses better for the eyes than eyeglasses?

A   The first contact lens was made in 1887. In the last one hundred years we've gone from a glass lens that hurt and frequently needed to be taken out of the eye to comfortable soft-plastic lenses. The soft contact was developed in Czechoslovakia in the late 1950s and was approved by the FDA in 1970. Today the FDA allows the selling of soft lenses that can remain in place day and night for up to thirty days. The use of these extended-wear lenses is controversial, however. People who wear them need to know the risks they are taking. Wearing soft contact lenses interferes with the ability of oxygen to get to the cornea. This reduced oxygen may be responsible for the increased incidence of corneal ulcers in extended-wear users. Dr. Walter Parkerson, an ophthalmologist from Charlotte, North Carolina, refuses to fit the extended-wear soft contact lens. He explains:

"The reason I do not fit extended wearers is two-fold. Number one, we have seen about sixteen corneal ulcers develop in patients wearing extended-wear contact lenses. Secondly, the medical literature is full of reports of people who developed corneal ulcers wearing extended-wear contact lenses, many of whom become legally blind. They had normal eyes prior to that time. So we do not desire our patients to live under the threat of having such a complication."

Ophthalmologists and optometrists are greatly concerned that contact lenses are now being sold in commercial establishments, such as drugstores and frame shops. It's important for lens wearers to fill their prescriptions where eye doctors are available to fit the lenses and to give follow-up cornea exams to the wearer two or three times a year.

The most serious problem of extended-wear use is the development of the pseudomonas infection in corneal ulcers. Pseudomonas can cause rapid melting-like destruction of the eye with perforation occurring within one to two days.

Dr. Parkerson says:

> Pseudomonas is the name of a bacteria. It's a gram-negative bacteria found in contaminated water or dirty contact-lens cases, dirty towels, and contaminated contact-lens solutions. When the bacteria involves the eye, it can cause a very severe corneal ulcer. It tends to involve the central part of the cornea where the visual axis is, and grows rapidly. If it's not treated immediately there's a great chance that the person would have permanent loss of vision.

These pseudomonas infections are rare. The incidence of pseudomonas in soft-contact-lens wearers, however, appears to be increasing. In a six-year study at Wills Eye Hospital in Philadelphia, more than half of the one hundred admissions for corneal ulcers occurred in the last eighteen months of the study. Although ulcerations and infections are more frequent with the extended-wear soft contact lens, they can occur with daily-wear soft contact lenses as well. Even when all doctors' instructions are followed diligently, patients have been known to suffer from pseudomonas infections.

Any acutely inflamed eye in a person wearing soft contact lenses should be treated as a medical emergency. Wearers should immediately remove the lens and store it in a moist container for later tests to determine what bacteria may have caused the problem. The patient should see an eye doctor immediately to be examined by a slit lamp, a special machine for examining the cornea.

Contact lenses are generally worn for cosmetic reasons. There are only a few eye problems in which contacts are necessary instead of glasses. Contacts were formerly used extensively after cataract surgery. But with the advent of an implantable intraocular lens, the need of contacts in post-op cataract patients has been nearly eliminated, except in very young children.

VISION PROBLEMS

Q   Is there any way to tell if my preschooler has trouble with his vision? He seems to squint a lot.

A   Your child may squint because he has lightly pigmented eyes, the lights are too bright for him, or he wants to see more clearly. There is a common misperception that young children cannot have their eyes and vision evaluated. Although a traditional eye chart examination may not be possible, mechanisms are available to determine how well a child sees. If your child prefers sedentary rather than active pastimes; squints often; is generally clumsy; or has difficulty catching, hitting, or throwing a ball, and you are concerned about his vision, it's probably time to seek professional advice.

Learning takes place through the senses, so good vision is one of a child's most valuable assets. Yet the eyes are vulnerable: nearly 100,000 eye injuries occur each year. Here are some tips for preserving your youngster's visual health at home.

1. Monitor TV viewing to minimize eye strain. A child should view TV from a distance of at least five times the width of the screen and in a room with soft overall lighting.

2. Be alert to danger signals of serious eye problems. Symptoms of serious trauma to the eye include blurred vision that does not clear with blinking, loss of all or part of the visual field, double vision, or a sharp stabbing or deep throbbing pain. The best first aid in such instances is to tape an eye shield, paper cup, or card-

board cone over the affected eye and transport the child to medical help.

3. Educate yourself in first aid for the eyes. For chemical burns of the eye, for example, wash the eye with water for five to twenty minutes, wipe any particles away from the face or hands, and transport the child (with eye uncovered this time) to medical help. Consult an ophthalmologist within twenty-four hours of the injury to have the eye examined.

RADIAL KERATOTOMY

Q I recently learned of a surgical procedure called radial keratotomy to correct problems of nearsightedness. I have worn glasses for years and would love to be able to toss them aside. How successful is this procedure?

A This controversial procedure to correct myopia was accidentally developed by a Russian ophthalmologist. A young patient of his was struck in the eye while wearing glasses. The glasses shattered, causing multiple superficial cuts onto the anterior layers of the front of the eye. When the bandages were removed, the young boy, to his surprise, could see without his glasses.

Thus the procedure known as radial keratotomy was developed. Eight to sixteen penetrating cuts, like spokes on a wheel, are made onto the cornea. The surgical procedure creates scars that shrink and make the front of the eye flatter, reducing the nearsightedness. (Nearsightedness is a condition where the patient's eye is too long or the front of the eye, the cornea, is too steep or curved so that the individual can see the objects nearby, but objects in the distance are blurred.)

If the cornea flattens too much, the patient will become farsighted and will need glasses. If the cornea does not flatten enough, the patient will be less nearsighted than before surgery. These patients may need to wear prescription lenses. At times the scars on the cornea prevent patients from wearing contact lenses.

Some ophthalmologists feel that the long-term risks will not be known for another decade or two, so anyone who can achieve satisfactory vision with glasses or contact lenses would be wise to continue using them until we know more about the long-term effects.

DENTAL HYGIENE

Q   My dentist says he won't wear gloves because he is allergic to latex. Isn't there some kind of requirement that dentists wear gloves?

A   All dentists should wear gloves as they work with their patients. No amount of washing can assure that all infectious viruses are killed. Two good reasons you should expect your dentist to wear gloves are patient-to-dentist transfer of viruses and dentist-to-patient transfer of viruses. The oral pathway is a common access for viruses.

An Indiana dentist recently gave up his dental practice because he had unwittingly spread hepatitis to six patients. Insurance companies in some states now require dentists and dental hygienists to use masks, gloves, and glasses when treating their patients in order to maintain their insurability. Dr. Edward Mitchell of the American Dental Association, told us, however, that recent surveys have shown that only 20 to 40 percent of dentists were using gloves. If your dentist isn't wearing gloves the next time you visit, ask him or her to do so. If the dentist doesn't comply, you should feel free to change dentists.

Studies have shown that dental personnel are five to ten times more likely than the general population to acquire hepatitis B. The dentist may not be aware of the exposure, because some hepatitis victims don't realize they have the disease. Periodontists and dentists often draw blood when they deep-clean and scale tartar from beneath the gums in their attempts to keep patients from losing teeth to periodontal disease. Thus they expose themselves to this blood-born infection.

DENTAL ILLNESS

Q   When I was a child, dental check-ups twice a year were routine in our family. As an adult, since I'm much less prone to cavities, I only make a trip to the dentist every three or four years, with satisfactory results. Is there any reason to go more often?

A   In addition to the maintenance of the health of your teeth and gums, your visits to the dentist have gained significance because of dentists' ability to diagnose systemic diseases early.

A dental examination is still the first line of defense against oral cancer. The dentists may notice white patches on the tongue or the insides of the cheek that are not easily removed. These are often precancerous. Even with regular care, it may be difficult to diagnose this disease, for the initial inflammation frequently disappears and leaves only a small growth.

You or your dentist may notice other warning signs of oral cancer, such as sores that bleed easily but do not heal, a lump or thickening in the mouth, or difficulty chewing, swallowing, or moving the tongue and the jaws. The checkup for oral cancer is especially important for those who use snuff or smokeless tobacco. Statistics from the National Cancer Institute indicate that users of these products are four times more likely to get cancers of the oral cavity and to have a fifty-fold increase in cancers of the cheek and gum.

A dental exam may discover diabetes. Periodontal disease (near or around the tooth) without an easily diagnosed reason, such as poor healing after surgery of the mouth or secondary infections such as candidiasis, may be indications of diabetes.

Some skin disorders may first become noticeable in the mouth. Lichen planus is a benign skin lesion generally thought to be the most common dermatological disease with oral manifestations. It often is noticed as white, scaly plaques inside the mouth. It is widely believed that there is a relationship between stress and the outbreak of symptoms.

A less common but potentially fatal skin lesion is called phemphigus; large blisters on the mucous membranes in the mouth are often the first indication of this disease. These blisters rupture easily and cause irregular erosions in the mouth.

Herpes simplex type I virus is often first seen by a dentist. Patients may have swelling and redness of the gums along with extremely painful eruptions of mucosa of the throat and mouth. A close cousin of the simplex, herpes zoster or shingles, may occasionally infect the nerves that service the mouth and throat. When this takes place, the initial presentation of the illness may be severe pain mimicking that of a toothache, with sores on one side of the mouth, cheek, or gums.

Vitamin deficiencies may also be diagnosed through careful assessment of the mouth during visits to your dentist. Folic acid deficiencies show up on a smooth, sore, reddened tongue. A person with B_{12} deficiency may have many of the same symptoms. Iron deficiencies cause the tongue to become smooth and sore, membranes to become pale, and ulcers to form.

This is only a partial list of the illnesses that can be found by regular dental checkups.

PREVENTING TOOTH DECAY

Q   How does a person keep teeth healthy?

A   The usual advice, which is still valid, is to brush after meals, floss daily, and have regular checkups and cleaning by a dentist. Adequate amounts of vitamin D and calcium, as well as flouridated water, have also traditionally been recommended.

Today, however, researchers are becoming more aware that other factors play a substantial role in a person's having healthy teeth and gums. For instance, the American Dental Association points out that smoking cigarettes, chewing tobacco, and dipping snuff are dangerous, because of the risks of oral cancer as well as the dangers to general periodontal health.

Those who smoke have greater accumulations of plaque and calculous in their mouths, leading directly to tooth decay and gum disease. Tobacco chewing and snuff dipping also increase plaque and calculus and cause cankers and other mouth irritations.

Consumption of sugar is another danger in maintaining healthy teeth. Sugar actually acts like an acid on teeth surfaces, and, like tobacco, promotes plaque and calculus.

On the positive side, there are some indications that vitamin C is an aid in the prevention of gum disease. A recent study using animals shows that vitamin C may have an effect on the gum tissue's resistance to disease. Vitamin C was found to prevent the scourge of scurvy more than a hundred years ago when bleeding gums were a common sign of this vitamin-C deficiency. The role of other nutrients, such as folic acid, calcium, and phosphorus, in the prevention and treatment of gum disease is also currently being studied.

Researchers say the preliminary indications are that vitamin C promotes the formation of collagen, an important protein found in connective tissue. Swollen and bleeding gums result from poorly formed collagen and can lead to pyorrhea, the leading cause of tooth loss.

Q   My son has just gotten his first two baby teeth. When should I take him to the dentist?

A   He'll be ready for his first trip to the dentist once he has all his baby molar teeth in the back of his mouth. These teeth can appear anywhere from nineteen to twenty-four months of age. Begin his dental care now by cleaning his teeth with gauze prior to sleep periods. As he grows older, use a soft-bristled toothbrush with a small amount of toothpaste after meals and before bed. Never allow your little one to fall asleep with a bottle or food in his mouth.

Q   What is the best way to save a knocked-out tooth?

A   You have probably heard of various ways to preserve a child's tooth while you are rushing him to the dentist. In the past, a favorite recommendation was to have the child hold the tooth in his mouth. If you have ever tried to persuade a screaming, frightened, bleeding child to do this, you know just how difficult it is. Now, scientists at the University of Florida have found that the best way to store the tooth is in milk. The ingredients in milk make it more likely that the tooth can be successfully implanted again. Since milk is usually available, it makes a convenient substance. So milk is good for the teeth in more ways than one!

Q   My dentist recommends that I have a root canal, but I have heard it's a painful procedure. I'm wondering if it wouldn't be better just to have the tooth extracted?

A   Most dentists agree that even a poorly done root canal is better than a good extraction, because the loss of a tooth causes so many problems: shifting of unequal pressures to other teeth, drifting of adjacent teeth toward the open space, or loss of bone because the jaw is now toothless in that spot.

EARDRUM TRANSPLANT

Q My daughter has had ear infections all her life. On a couple of occasions she has had a punctured eardrum and drainage from her ear. For the past eight months she has had a distinct hearing impairment in her right ear. Is she likely to remain hard of hearing, or are there any new medical discoveries that could help her problem?

A If she has a chronically perforated eardrum, she may need an eardrum transplant. Although this operation has not had the extensive national press coverage accorded organ transplants, doctors in Europe and in California—where researchers have experimented with various methods of storing eardrums—have been performing the surgery since the mid-1960s with a 70 to 80 percent success rate.

More recently, an otologist in Palo Alto, California, has transplanted eardrums that had been prepared and stored in a buffered formaldehyde solution. This solution seems to strengthen the eardrum and also ensures its sterility. There have been reperforations in only a small percentage of cases and no evidence of rejection. This technique has proved extremely helpful in restoring hearing cases where the eardrum and little ear bones have been damaged by chronic infections such as your daughter's.

To bring the benefits of this development to as many as possible, Project Hear, a nonprofit medical foundation for ear research, was established with the aid of a grant from the John A. Hartford Foundation. Project Hear is developing an eardrum-bank program with regional banks, much like the national eye-bank program. It's primary purpose is to make eardrums available to ear surgeons all over the country. Anyone wishing to donate his eardrums or those of his deceased relatives may now do so. The eardrum tissue must be removed within twenty-four hours after death.

Other factors such as scarring of the eardrum, damage to the bones of the middle ear, fluid retention or tissue overgrowth in the middle ear could also be playing a role in your daughter's hearing impairment. Because of the number of possibilities, it is imperative that you have a complete audiological evaluation done immediately. Once the cause has been determined, then the appropriate treatment can be prescribed.

HEARING LOSS IN CHILDREN

Q   My child seems to be an expert at ignoring me when I speak to her. On the other hand, I sometimes suspect that she may have a hearing loss. What signs would indicate that she is not just tuning me out?

A   Common clues indicating that a child needs a hearing test are the child's turning the TV set volume louder and louder or not responding to commands. Watch the situations when your child ignores you. Children do focus on their toys or games and do not always respond to common interruptions when they are busy. Children also have a way of not hearing undesirable requests. However, if your youngster misses "fun" conversations (does she hear the ice cream truck but miss your call to come in from play?), has trouble hearing while on the telephone, misunderstands similar sounding words, please see your doctor or arrange for a hearing test.

Typically, a child with a conductive loss in the middle ear will speak more softly, unlike an older person with a nerve hearing loss, who will speak more loudly.

If your school system doesn't have a simple test program to screen for early hearing loss, you might want to help organize one.

Q   Several of my family members have experienced difficulty with their hearing as they have grown older. What are some suggestions to prevent deafness?

131

A   Hearing loss is the most common chronic physical disability in the United States. However, because it often occurs slowly, most people do not realize their degree of hearing loss until it becomes serious.

To prevent it, here are some situations of which to be aware:

- Noise: Blood flow to hair cells in the ear is reduced by blood vessel spasms during exposure to loud noises. Scar tissue is formed, which replaces the live cells. Shock-wave damage increases as noises grow louder and longer. Cordless telephones can create noise damage. Individuals have suffered hearing loss from the ringer in the earpiece of the cordless phones. Most manufacturers have now taken the ringer out of the earpiece. If you have a cordless phone, make sure it doesn't ring in your ear.
- Cigarette smoking: Like noise, it decreases the amount of blood flow to the hair cells in the inner ear.
- Diet: Atherosclerosis is thought to be a frequent cause of age-related hearing loss. We urge our readers to exercise and to switch to a diet low in fat and high in soluble fiber, hoping that hearing loss can thus be curbed or even reversed.
- Drugs: Several common drugs, such as high doses of aspirin, are toxic to the ears. If, while taking any drugs, you develop any hearing-related symptoms such as ringing or deafness, consult your physician immediately.
- Otospongiosis: A hereditary disease, otospongiosis causes an abnormal growth in the inner ear. This condition usually develops in persons between the ages of 15 and 50 and in women more than in men. Surgery can dramatically help lessen this hearing loss if done early enough.

An old rule is that if you think you or someone you live with has a hearing problem, you are probably right.

Take time to answer the following questions if you suspect you are losing your hearing:

- Do you feel that people mumble?
- Do people consistently talk too softly?
- Do you place the volume on the radio and television higher than is comfortable for those around you?
- Do you often ask for things to be repeated (or pretend you heard to avoid asking)?
- Do you habitually turn one ear toward the person who is speaking?
- Do you hear ringing or buzzing sounds in your head?
- Have you experienced episodes of dizziness?

If you suspect you have impaired hearing, the best way to find out is to see an audiologist or an otorhinolaryngologist (ENT doctor) for a hearing test.

Hearing loss can cause personality changes and even paranoia. Far better to hear what people are saying about you than to imagine it!

HEARING AIDS

Q The doctor has suggested I be fitted for a hearing aid, but I am hesitating because of my memories of my grandfather's struggles with his hearing aid. Have there been any new developments in hearing aid technology?

A When Helen Keller was asked which was the greater handicap, deafness or blindness, she responded, to everyone's surprise, "deafness." Doctors know that deafness has a more damaging effect on the personality than does blindness.

If you had had a chance to listen in on grandpa's hearing aid a generation ago, you would have found that most of the sounds were unintelligible and irritating. The aid made everything louder, especially the noises we have learned to disregard. The hapless users had to learn to "hear" all over again. The old hearing aids were a far cry from the sophisticated, micro, all-in-the-ear hearing devices available today.

Normally hearing involves the movement of three tiny bones or ossicles in the middle ear, commonly called the hammer, the anvil, and the stirrup. Sometimes these tiny bones have been damaged by infection or injury, or the foot plate of the stirrup bone may have grown solid to the bone of the snail-shaped cochlea, a condition called otosclerosis. Otosclerosis is now treated surgically and the tiny bone is replaced by a piece of plastic.

Sometimes the tiny bones in the ear produce what is called conductive hearing losses. In these circumstances, the hearing organ (the cochlea) and the hearing nerve are still able to function if only the sound can be brought to them. Most hearing losses, fortunately, are of this type. For those with conductive hearing problems, hearing aids can be of great value.

Hearing is sometimes lost as a result of failure of the hearing nerves due to blood circulation problems such as atherosclerosis, viral infections of nerves, such as shingles, or destruction of the nerve by a tumor. Deafness that is a result of the failure of the cochlea or of the auditory nerve is called nerve deafness.

Acquiring a hearing aid under these conditions is like fixing the telephone after the wire has been cut. Thus older people are sometimes hoodwinked when buying hearing aids. Go first to an otologist, or ear physician, who does not sell hearing aids. An otologist can tell you what type of hearing loss you have and whether a hearing aid would be of any value, without any conflict of interest.

It is important, too, for a partially deaf person to try out a hearing aid before committing to buy it.

Advanced electronics makes possible new "smart" hearing aids. These devices selectively amplify only the tones involved in speech communication. By suppressing noise frequencies, these smart hearing aids actually help replace the function of selective hearing that the person has lost. Another amazing feature of these miniature marvels is that they are tiny enough to be concealed within the ear itself.

Hearing aids aren't just for the elderly. A one-day-old baby can be tested for hearing, and it is not unusual to fit a six-month-old baby with a hearing aid. This often prevents the child from being branded a slow learner, as it greatly improves the hearing-impaired youngster's ability to speak and learn.

Reported cases of hearing loss are increasing for a number of reasons. People are living longer. Blasts of rock music are hurting youngsters' ears, which will cause hearing loss at a much earlier age. Noises from lawn mowers, chain saws, and other loud machines can be harmful. Use ear plugs when you must be exposed to a loud noise over a period of time, especially in confined quarters, or when you are near noisy jets, motorboats, tractors, or any loud power equipment.

Don't miss out on the sounds around you because of a past experience. Call today and set up an evaluation.

EAR INFECTIONS

Q My child had several ear infections last winter. At the time he was six to nine months old. What causes this problem, and why is it so rampant among babies?

A Children have more ear infections than adults because their Eustachian tubes are short and narrow. This tube connects the middle ear to the back of the throat, above the tonsils and behind the nose. If a child has a cold, this tube becomes plugged and no air can get into the middle ear. Fluid fills the middle ear so it does not transmit sound well. That's why children with middle ear infections or fluid have decreased hearing, as well as pain and fever. Children also have more ear infections than adults because they are more prone to have colds.

Q   I have ringing in my ears just as my mother had when she was about my age. I remember her doctor told her it was due to high blood pressure; however, I do not have high blood pressure. What else could be causing this ringing? At times it is louder than others.

A   I would suggest that you have an audiogram test—a series of tones used to determine one's hearing loss—administered by an ear, nose, and throat (ENT) specialist. Ringing in the ears (tinnitus) is often associated with a hearing loss in the 4000 cps (cycles per second) range or above. The normal hearing range for speech is 500 to 2000 cps. Typical speech volume needs to be at a level of 40 decibels (db) for a minimum acceptable level and usually is closer to 60 db in normal conversation.

Exposure to excessive noise may be the single most common contributing factor to this high-frequency hearing loss. Working around loud machinery, shooting guns, driving loud equipment, and listening to loud music can cause noise trauma. Infections such as meningitis, encephalitis, and head injury may also contribute to hearing loss. Some drugs (aspirin and streptomycin) when used in excess may cause ringing in the ears.

High blood pressure may play a role in some cases of tinnitus, but even more important than the actual high blood pressure itself is the condition that often accompanies high blood pressure in the middle-aged and older group—the build-up of cholesterol plaques in the vessels that supply the inner ear.

Pressure changes in the fluid in the inner ear may give the sensation of a change in the volume of the ringing.

During a person's working or waking hours, background noise is often at a sufficient level that the tinnitus goes relatively unnoticed. But at bedtime, when the background noise is greatly reduced, the tinnitus can become very annoying. Bringing in some low-level background noise, such as music or radio static, will often help such a person get to sleep.

People who have tinnitus should avoid further noise trauma, because this can worsen an already unpleasant problem.

CHAPTER 8

Cancer Consciousness

Cancer ruthlessly strikes at least one member of nearly every family in the United States. It is one of the most feared diseases to befall an individual. And while researchers continue their efforts to find cures, early detection, good nutrition, physical fitness, mental well-being are presently the factors most likely to allow a person to recover from cancer's insidious intrusion.

The following questions and answers offer information on numerous types of cancers and suggestions for cancer prevention and early detection.

SKIN CANCER

Q   How serious are skin cancers? What are the early warning signs?

A   On women like Liz Taylor, moles are called beauty marks. But innocent "beauty marks" should be looked upon with suspicion if they change in size, color, texture, or even if they begin to itch. Moles that begin to thicken, become red around the edges, tingle or spread could become malignant and thus, deadly. If you find a mole changing in any way, you should act quickly: prompt treatment can be life saving.

Malignant melanomas account for ninety percent of all deaths from skin cancer. Most skin cancers are not lethal, but this one is fast-moving and dangerous. When treated early, ninety percent of malignant melanomas can be cured. If, however, treatment is not begun until after metastasis (the cancer spreading through the bloodstream to distant sites), the five-year survival rate drops to less than ten percent.

BREAST CANCER

Q At what age should I have my first mammogram for breast cancer? I am thirty-four. My mother had one of her breasts removed about fifteen years ago (her health is good now), so I know I am in a high-risk category.

A A baseline mammogram is recommended for women at the age of thirty-five. Women who are forty to forty-nine years of age and who are at increased risk for breast cancer should have mammograms yearly, as should all women who are fifty years of age and older.

For women who discover their own breast lumps, the average life span after that is seven years for white women and four years for black women. On the other hand, if a lump is discovered before it is palpable, in a screening program such as mammography and ultrasound, the life expectancy is almost normal. Unfortunately 90 percent of breast cancers are discovered by the women themselves.

The chances of five-year survival are far greater if a breast cancer is discovered early by a routine mammogram. If a tumor is caught early, the breast does not necessarily have to be removed; lumpectomy is a good option. Betty Ford, Happy Rockefeller, Shirley Temple Black, Nancy Reagan, and many other women are living proof that there is life after breast cancer. Your chances of being counted among the fortunate are much better if you go for your first mammogram at the age of thirty-five. You and your doctor can determine a schedule for repeated exams.

The five-year survival rate is greater than 85 percent when the cancer is discovered while very small, but less than 35 percent when the cancer is not diagnosed until after it has spread from the breast into the lymph nodes. Breast tumors only one-tenth of a centimeter in size (that's the size of a pinhead) can be seen by x-ray long before they can be felt. Most lumps are about one centimeter or almost half an inch when they can be palpated. By physical examination alone, it's almost impossible to detect a small tumor growing within large breasts.

Since new cancer prevention guidelines recommend women over the age of fifty have yearly mammograms, low-dose radiation is important. Other guidelines to follow include giving yourself a monthly breast exam, having palpation of the breasts by qualified medical personnel on an annual basis, and having a baseline x-ray mammogram at the age of thirty-five. The good news about breast cancer screening is that newer x-ray mammography equipment now gives far less radiation than previous machines. Ask questions about the amount of radiation to which you will be exposed when you undergo mammography because the new low-dose equipment gives about 1 percent of the radiation of the older equipment that is still being used in some hospitals.

Because ultrasound has no radiation and is not known to have any risks, all women can benefit from the use of this screening device—not instead of, but in addition to the national guidelines for mammography. Breast ultrasound is now available in an estimated one hundred medical centers throughout the United States.

CERVICAL CANCER

Q   What measures can be taken to prevent cancer of the cervix? After my last child was born, the doctor found (through a Pap smear) some dysplasia on my cervix. These irregularities were removed through a biopsy and conization. Should I be worried about the onset of cervical cancer?

A   Mounting evidence suggests that cervical cancer is an infectious sexually transmitted disease. Some researchers believe that in addition to herpes, the human papillomavirus, which causes the growth of a flat genital wart called a condyloma, may be involved in causing this cancer. Risk factors include becoming sexually active at an early age, having multiple sexual partners, and having a sexually transmitted disease.

Of the 8,000 women who will die this year from cancer of the cervix, virtually 100 percent of them will have been previously exposed to the genital strain of herpes. In addition, women with sexually transmitted venereal warts, or condylomas, have 1200 to 2000 times greater risk of getting cervical cancer than women without a condyloma.

As you can see, a frequent Pap smear is much more important for some women than for others. A woman who has genital herpes or a condyloma should have a Pap smear twice a year. It is a well-known fact that women with genital herpes have seven times the risk of cervical cancer than average. And a woman whose husband has had multiple sex partners is also at higher risk.

Other researchers feel that the herpes simplex virus involves a "hit and run" mechanism that can induce the changes in cells that cause them to become tumors. Thereafter, the cells remain transformed in the absence of any detectable herpes virus.

Dr. Gerard Nuovo at Columbia University told us that their research has shown overwhelming evidence that papillomaviruses 16 and 18 cause cervical cancer. He told us that papillomaviruses 6 and 11 behave very differently and do not go on to become cancerous lesions. He has been working in the Columbia University laboratory of Dr. Ralph Richart, whose innovative work has led us to recognize cervical cancer as a sexually transmitted cancer.

Dr. Norman Dahm, a gynecologist who treats papillomaviruses and cervical cancer, reported one case history of a girl who had gone from a negative Pap smear to a full-blown, advanced stage-3 cancer of the cervix in nine months.

"The American Cancer Society guidelines should be stiffened, because a patient can go from a negative Pap smear to invasive cancer in less than a year," Dr. Dahm says. This information that Dr. Richart and his colleagues have gathered through studying human papillomaviruses has tremendous value.

This human papillomavirus is probably the first true oncogenic virus or cocarcinogen that we've been able to study. And because of it, patients right now have a much shorter transit time—that is, they can go from a negative Pap smear to cancer of the cervix in a very short period of time. I doesn't take 20 years. We can't tell patients that anymore.

At this time, because we're seeing so many patients at a young age and because sexual activity is started at such a young age, it's even more important to do Pap smears on these young women. Often the mother will say, 'When should my daughter have the Pap smear?' Every patient should have a Pap smear as soon as she becomes sexually active. If a patient has two negative Pap smears, it does not mean she doesn't need a Pap smear every year.

In countries where females become sexually active at an early age, women report cases of cervical cancer at a younger age. Historically, it was a disease women developed in their thirties and forties. Now physicians are beginning to see women in their twenties with cervical cancer.

"We try to get women to come in often, and if they're at high risk, every six months isn't too often," Dr. Dahm says. "If their husbands are giving them papillomaviruses, you have to get their husbands treated. I tell these women to check the penis with a magnifying glass. The urologist would also stain the penis with acetic acid or vinegar to locate the lesions. If they see even tiny condylomatous warts anywhere, the husband can be treated just as simply with freezing or with laser."

Researchers estimate that there will be 12,800 new cases of cervical cancer this year and that 6,800 women will die from cervical cancer. Avoidance of risk factors and adherence to the suggested guidelines for Pap smears is the best hope for diminishing these numbers.

Q   How accurate are the tests that are used to detect cancer in the early stages?

A   Although generally accurate, under certain conditions some tests give misleading results. For example, the stool test—the examination of a stool sample for hidden blood, an indication of possible colon cancer—can give false negative results if the patient has been taking vitamin C.

The bottom line is this: When you have a stool test, go off vitamin C first, no matter what test you or your doctor uses. Millions of Americans over thirty years of age take more than 250 mg of vitamin C daily, so if they were to take a stool test their results could be inaccurate.

Women can also have a *false negative* if they douche or bathe prior to a Pap smear. This causes the test to fail to disclose abnormal cells.

False positive tests, on the other hand, are also common. Aspirin, vitamin B, vitamin A, iron preparations, large amounts of caffeine, vaginal douching powders, cold remedies, and laxatives can all trigger false positives.

Q   Can you explain flexible sigmoidoscopy?

A   Flexible sigmoidoscopy is one of the best tests for early discovery of a malignancy in the rectum or colon, yet far too few people have taken advantage of it.

The fiberoptic sigmoidoscope follows the curvature of the colon easily, causing little discomfort when your doctor does this examination. Furthermore, it can be advanced farther into the colon to look for polyps or other diseases.

Eighty-three percent of cancers of the colon and a high percentage of noncancerous polyps can be seen by sigmoidoscopy, and a sample can actually be taken through these instruments to confirm diagnosis.

Cancer of the colon is the second most common cancer (lung cancer being the most common). A positive screening test for occult blood often precipitates a sigmoidoscopy, especially in those people who do not regularly visit their physician for routine physical exams. This leads to earlier diagnosis and a higher rate of cure for this cancer. Routine sigmoidoscopy is a part of the health maintenance protocol for men and women over fifty, even if stool tests for occult blood are negative.

LARYNX, LUNG, AND ESOPHAGEAL CANCER

Q   Why is it important to have one's larynx and vocal cords checked?

A   Not every malignant polyp is obliging enough to develop on a vocal cord, thus causing hoarseness, an early warning sign of cancer. A large percentage of cancers of the larynx develop above or below the larynx and grow silently for long periods before producing symptoms. Every patient should have these hidden areas of the throat examined, especially when he has symptoms of polyps. Tumors in the pharynx and larynx hold promise of a high rate of cure if found and treated early. But the prognosis for neglected growths is poor.

If you are a moderate to heavy smoker and drinker, it is especially imperative that you have a physician examine your larynx. Between 95 and 99 percent of laryngectomy patients needing their voice box removed have been smokers *and* drinkers. In a recent poll for The Saturday Evening Post Society, we asked the question, *"If you smoke and drink alcoholic beverages*, have you had your vocal cords visualized by a physician?" More than half, or 285 out of 507 respondents, said that their cords had *never* been examined.

For more than a hundred years, the angled mirror, which was technically difficult to handle, was the only office tool available for doctors to use to see the larynx and surrounding tissue. The expertise and skill required to use the mirror made it difficult for the typical general physician to employ. So by default, he left its use to the trained otorhinolaryngologist, or ear, nose, and throat specialist.

Fortunately, Japanese and American technology has created new equipment that does a splendid job of showing the larynx and revealing with great accuracy any polyps, even below the vocal cords. A new right-angle telescope, called a LarynxVue, has been developed for use by the primary physician. Even though untrained in the mirror technique, the physician can see the larynx clearly, with great ease and speed, making it feasible to include this procedure as part of routine exams. For the throat specialist, the fiber-optic laryngoscope, which is hardly larger than a shoe string and can be put through the nostril with only a very mild local anesthetic, has been created. Both the family practitioner and the specialist can now diagnose early signs of cancer.

Q What are the earliest steps a physician can take to diagnose lung cancer?

A Some of you may remember when Pap smears first became available. Doctors were enthusiastic because they knew the new test would cut down cervical cancer deaths to a fraction of what they had been.

A few researchers and clinicians now believe that getting so-called "lung" Pap smears is just as important, especially for people who are heavy smokers. The smears are taken from samples of coughed-up sputum.

One advocate of the pulmonary Pap smear is Dr. Robert J. Ginsberg, chief of thoracic surgery at Mt. Sinai Hospital in Toronto, Canada. In a presentation to the University of Toronto medical faculty, he reported that in his experience, 100 percent of patients were cured of their lung tumors when the tiny cancers were identified by cytology while too small to be seen on x-ray. The tumors were localized and surgically removed.

Dr. Ginsberg urges smokers over forty-five years of age to be screened annually by sputum cytology and chest x-ray for the remainder of their lives.

The lung Pap smear is very simple for the patient. Sputum is collected first thing in the morning on three consecutive mornings. The patient preserves the cells by storing the sputum in a container of alcohol, then mailing the specimen to a laboratory for examination. The interpretation of the cell residue is best done by a laboratory with much experience in reading and interpreting pulmonary cytology.

Dr. Geno Saccomanno of St. Mary's Hospital in Grand Junction, Colorado, has discovered lung cancers years before they are large enough to cast a shadow on an x-ray. He began more than thirty years ago examining cells coughed up by uranium miners and smokers. He believes that use of cytology can reveal tumors about three years sooner than a chest x-ray. Discovering lung cancer years before it shows on an x-ray gives surgeons an infinitely better chance of curing the disease than they have after the tumor has grown and spread.

Q   Even though I have smoked for many years, I don't seem to have any signs of developing emphysema. Why should I bother to quit now?

A "Give us this day our daily breath" is the plea, conscious or unconscious, of more than a million people in this country who suffer from emphysema. Testing for emphysema is a most neglected area of medicine. Smokers who smugly say, "I just came from the doctor and have a clean bill of health," haven't any reason to feel complacent. They simply don't realize the many limitations of a general physical exam in which the doctor may x-ray the lungs, but rarely does the doctor check the primary function of the lungs—*breathing*. Unless a smoker has had a spirometry test of his or her lung capacity, there may be no obvious evidence that emphysema has begun to work havoc with the lungs. I think the spirometer is so important that large corporations should install them in their companies' physical fitness departments.

Surprisingly, insurance companies, which often require blood pressure data, don't require spirometry tests, which simply measure lung function. Spirometers can pick up early signs of lung diseases in people in their twenties, thirties, and forties in time for a lifestyle change to be most beneficial.

The test is easy to take and inexpensive. First you breathe deeply, then exhale forcefully into a tube connected to the spirometer. The machine measures the amount or volume of air exhaled and can show what structures of the lung are damaged as well as how much air is retained in the lung. Some sophisticated spirometers also give information about your lungs as you inspire, or breathe in.

All of us lose lung capacity beginning around age twenty, but most of us have been blessed with far more than we will ever need and will never notice the deficit. However, some smokers begin to lose lung function quite early, and we know these individuals will continue to lose lung function at an accelerated rate. By middle age, these persons will have incapacitating emphysema. If no testing occurs before a smoker reaches age fifty, too much tissue will have been destroyed; quitting will help, but severe damage will have been done.

The tissue in your lungs, if stretched out, can cover two tennis courts. The normal lung is solid in appearance, but in each lung the tissue is actually made of 100 million tiny sacs called alveoli. In these air sacs oxygen is absorbed and carbon dioxide is removed from the bloodstream. In emphysema these alveoli break down, creating a Swiss-cheese or lacy appearance in the lung. The elasticity of the lung is lost, and much like an overstretched balloon, the lung no longer releases all the air. The air sacs hold more stale air trapped in ever-enlarging pockets in the lungs. Adequate amounts of oxygen can't get in and carbon dioxide can't get out, creating "air hunger," the panicky feeling of suffocation typical of severe, advanced emphysema.

The changes brought about by emphysema occur steadily over 15 to 25 years. They cannot be seen on chest x-rays until the lungs are significantly and permanently damaged. The physician cannot hear early changes when listening for breathing sounds. Slight shortness of breath when exercising is usually explained as poor physical conditioning or the aging process.

A recent study at Harvard has shown that smoking has an especially devastating effect on teen-agers by preventing their lungs from achieving their full growth. A teen-ager who has smoked for two and a half years will have a 10 percent loss in development of normal vital capacity. Five years of teen-age smoking brings a 15 percent loss.

If you smoke, ask your doctor for a spirometry test. If you have a smoker in your family, urge the smoker not only to have a spirometry test, but also to request an alpha-1 antitrypsin test to know whether this enzyme deficiency exists. If it does, there is an 80 to 90 percent chance of the relative developing emphysema, if he or she continues to smoke.

Q My husband has been trying to quit smoking. He uses an air filter that he thinks cuts down on the smoke, but lately I've insisted that he smoke outside. As a mother of three young children, I worry about the effects of second-hand smoke. Is there any recent information about this?

A Spouses as well as children of smokers risk side effects from second-hand or passive smoke including eye, nose, and throat irritations, lung disease, and cancer. The Department of Health and Human Services and the Environmental Protection Agency found that non-smoking spouses of smokers had a 30 percent rise in lung cancer. Children of smokers developed more bronchitis, pneumonia, and other respiratory infections; had more chronic ear infections; and also risked impaired lung development, stunted growth (a pregnant woman's child is also at risk for this through second-hand smoke), and lung disease later in life. Although air filters do reduce eye, nose, and throat irritation, there is no guarantee that the disease-causing substances are eliminated. It is also discouraging to note that children of smokers are more likely to smoke cigarettes than children of nonsmokers.

Children should not have to be exposed to the harmful effects of cigarette smoke, and it shouldn't be possible for children or teen-agers to buy tobacco products. We want to get cigarettes under the counters and not permit them to be sold in unattended, unsupervised vending machines.

We asked Surgeon General C. Everett Koop what concerned persons could do about the smoking problem.

They have to become educated. They have to recognize that smoking is a problem and it's a health problem. It's not just a nasty habit. Nicotine is an addictive drug. In fact, the National Institute on Drug Abuse has said *it is the most addictive drug in our society.* And then they have to decide whether or not their priorities of health for themselves, their families, and indeed, for the nation are high enough that they are willing to do something about it.

Although the evidence has increasingly pointed to the harmful effects of smoking on smokers and non-smokers alike, the tobacco industry has continued to pour millions of dollars into ad campaigns designed to promote smoking. To counteract this, numerous groups have been formed to help decrease smoking by publishing studies highlighting the dangers of tobacco, lobbying for the antismoking laws, promoting higher taxes on tobacco products, calling for tougher warnings on cigarette packs, and pushing for restricting or banning the use of tobacco on public property.

Q   I have warned my son countless times that chewing tobacco is as hazardous to his health as smoking cigarettes. But he insists upon chewing tobacco because it fits with his "image" and the advertising he sees in the media doesn't help back me up.

A   Tobacco manufacturers are undertaking a major campaign to promote the use of smokeless tobacco. Smokeless tobacco comes in three forms: chewing tobacco; dry snuff, which is usually inhaled; and moist snuff, called dip, which is tucked between the gum and lip.

Unlike smoking, snuff dipping and tobacco chewing have traditionally been limited to a small percentage of the population located mainly in the South. Sports personalities and entertainers, however, have transformed a habit once thought to be dirty and unsociable into a practice viewed as a status symbol with teen-agers.

It is deplorable to take advantage of young people by getting them addicted to a dangerous drug before they are mature enough to know better. Recently a shredded bubble gum packaged just like pink shredded tobacco appeared on the market. Even the offers on the back for sports equipment are similar. All the better to lure children. Sports figures extol smokeless tobacco on television to convert the youngsters who are trying to emulate the macho look of their heroes.

Studies conducted in Louisiana in 1983 found that 21 percent of ten-year-olds in Louisiana were dipping snuff. Rhonda Atkins from Oklahoma City was horrified when she found her five-year-old son had been using snuff obtained from a neighborhood food store. The grocer told her there was not a law against it, so she campaigned to set an age limit for tobacco purchase, which has now become law in Oklahoma.

The case of Sean Marsee of Oklahoma shocked the public into scrutinizing this dangerous habit.

Sean, a star member of his school's track team, voted most outstanding athlete of the year 1983, had been addicted to snuff from the age of twelve.

He developed what he thought was a cold sore on his tongue, but a biopsy showed that it was actually a malignant tumor. In the first operation a few days after his high school graduation in 1983, the doctors removed one-third of Sean's tongue. Other, more extensive, operations followed until his death in 1984.

Q I have heard that the occurrence of esophageal cancer, one of the worst kinds of cancer, has been related to the deficiency of a trace metal in a person. Has any research been done to substantiate this?

A The outlook for a patient with esophageal cancer is grim indeed. Even in the cases of early detection, only five of one hundred victims survive five years.

Dr. S.P. Yang and his associates at Texas Tech University have done some exciting new work on this type of cancer, however. Their data indicated that the trace metal molybdenum is a key to preventing this usually fatal disease. Sufficient molybdenum in the diet may prevent people from acquiring this form of cancer.

In the U. S., the incidence of esophageal cancer is 13.3 per 100,000 black males and 3.5 per 100,000 white males. It is twice as common in males as in females. In our country the most common association with cancer of the esophagus is with cigarette smoking and excessive alcohol intake. However, it must be remembered that persons with these combined habits generally practice poor nutrition from the standpoint of vitamin and mineral intake.

A common denominator of all the high-risk population is the exposure of the lining of the esophagus to carcinogens, whether it is cigarette smoke, alcohol, nitrosamines, or viruses.

If your well water contains deficient amounts of molybdenum or if you eat large amounts of homegrown vegetables and you're unsure whether there is molybdenum in the soil, take a dietary supplement containing molybdenum and other trace minerals.

Q   I felt painfully alone when I learned that I had a rare form of malignant lymphoma. Do you have any advice for ways to cope with this devastating news?

A   The response to the sudden diagnosis of cancer is often a mixture of anger, denial, despair, and hope. The hope comes from the faith that God is with us, which yields the courage and the will for healing and makes it possible to accept the difficult and often painful path that may be necessary for treatment and cure. You need the faith and determination to search out the best possible treatment for your disease: Knowledge is an important coping mechanism. Please ask questions and try to understand the changes that have occurred.

When a doctor informs a patient that he or she has cancer, the patient should ask the doctor if he has frequently treated cancer patients and what type of cancer he has treated. The patient has the right to decide who cares for him throughout his illness and to expect a high level of expertise. Most physicians understand this need and can assist in choosing a physician who has expertise and is geographically close to the patient. The doctor can telephone the National Cancer Institute for PDQ, Physician's Data Query, a computerized data-base developed by the Cancer Institute that can help find names of oncologists and their specialties. Or patients and families can call 1-800-4-CANCER. The staff of the National Cancer Institute will respond to any inquiries by referring to various resources, including PDQ.

Dr. Vincent DeVita, director of the NCI, can be thanked for promoting the PDQ program. Dr. DeVita pointed out that when a patient is diagnosed with cancer and faces the possibility of losing his or her life, the patient should not be shy about hurting the doctor's feelings. The patient has a responsibility to get the best medical care possible. So if you have a rare or unusual cancer, tell your doctor you want to go to someone with experience treating such cancers.

————————CHAPTER 9————————

Safety Tips and Emergency Procedures

Safety precautions work in much the same way as good nutrition. They are "preventive medicine" for numerous accidents and infirmities. Of course, no environment is 100 percent accident-proof, and mishaps will befall even the most conscientious person. When accidents or emergencies do occur, it is important to be ready to act in a responsible way to help the victim, whether it's you or someone else.

FOOD POISONING

Q   I've heard it's not uncommon to get food poisoning from turkey. What precautions need to be taken in preparing this favorite holiday bird?

A   Let me illustrate with a story: Each Thanksgiving a doting mother baked a large turkey and invited all her married sons and their families for a feast. She was a marvelous cook and most of the guests ate the delicious turkey and dressing.

Each year, the day after Thanksgiving, family members returned to their respective homes and became ill with the flu. They suffered diarrhea, upset stomachs, fatigue, and achiness. But it wasn't the flu at all. What was it?

They were suffering from food poisoning. The stuffing, which had been prepared the day before Thanksgiving and put in the turkey's cavity, was found teeming with salmonella. Salmonella bacteria are common inhabitants (in small numbers) of the carcasses of chickens and turkeys. When they are permitted to multiply rapidly, they cause food poisoning.

In a large turkey it is difficult to heat the innermost portions of the dressing, so the dressing provides an excellent culture medium for rapid breeding of salmonella. The center of the turkey should be heated to 180°F. Heat hamburger to 170°F to kill salmonella. Because the salmonella are tasteless and odorless, it is impossible to identify them before ingestion.

Another type of bacteria that causes food poisoning is *staphylococcus*. Between 20 and 50 percent of healthy people normally carry staph germs on their hands and in their nasal passages. This bacteria can be carried by flies or even be airborne in dust. It takes a million of these organisms for each gram of food to make a person ill, yet in only a few hours, under favorable conditions, they can multiply to this number.

When food is left at room temperature or above, the staph multiply and release toxic substances. Staph contamination occurs most often in foods containing mayonnaise such as macaroni and potato salads, deviled eggs, sandwiches, and some seafood dishes. Avoid foods at buffets or on picnics if sufficient refrigeration or adequate heating is not available. Also, if previously contaminated foods have enough toxin, simple reheating will not make the foods safe. In addition, foods, once cooked, should not be left to cool slowly.

Botulism poisoning, which is much more serious, occurs less frequently than staph contamination. *Cholstridium botulinum* produces spores that release toxins, which are transported by the blood to the nerve endings. There they can affect such vital processes as swallowing and breathing. Boiling for ten minutes or using a pressure cooker at 240°F can destroy the toxin. The spores in themselves are not harmful, but as they germinate, they release toxins that are lethal.

Home-canned foods are the foods most likely to cause botulism, particularly canned corn and beans because of their low acidity. Peas, meats, fish, and poultry are also in this problem group.

Spinach, asparagus, beets, and pumpkins are less likely to be problems because they have medium acidity. If in doubt, boil them before eating. Most tomatoes, pears, and red cabbages are sufficiently acidic to inhibit toxins.

Botulism is more poisonous than both cyanide and the deadliest snake venom. Swollen bottle lids and can ends indicate its presence. If a jar looks suspicious, never taste even the smallest morsel—throw it out.

After ingestion, the incubation time for botulism is 12 to 36 hours. Then the victim develops nausea, vomiting, blurred vision, swallowing difficulties, slurred speech, a dry mouth, and breathing difficulties. Constipation occurs rather than diarrhea. Botulism poisoning requires emergency hospitalization and treatment with botulinum antitoxin. If this condition is suspected, take the possibly contaminated food or a portion of the vomitus to the hospital for testing.

Q   I have heard that babies can get very sick from eating honey.

A   Honey may contain the bacterial spores that can cause infant botulism. The American Academy of Pediatrics and the Centers for Disease Control recommend that infants younger than twelve months of age not be fed honey, in order to reduce the risk of infant botulism.

Although the disease is rare, it is a very serious one affecting the nervous system. Since the disease in infants was first diagnosed, more than 500 cases have been reported in the United States. An estimated one out of five babies who developed the disease had been fed honey.

Some of the symptoms include

• a healthy baby not strong enough to suck or cry as usual;

- a weakening of the baby's arms or legs;
- a weakness of the neck in which the baby's head becomes floppy.

Often, severe constipation occurs before or after such weakness. Infants who develop this disease have a good prognosis with hospitalization and proper treatment.

To help avoid infant botulism do not add honey to your baby's food, water, or formula; do not dip your baby's pacifier in honey; and do not give your baby any honey as medicine. Children older than one year of age are able to safely ingest honey.

POISONING: PREVENTION AND CARE

Q One of my greatest fears is that my child will consume a poisonous substance I will have carelessly left around the house. What should I do in the event of this emergency?

A Every year, an estimated 3 million accidental poisonings occur in our country, many of them involving small children. Youngsters are naturally curious, so it is the responsibility of adults to protect them from the medications and cleaning agents that might harm them. Store all poisonous household cleansers and all medications out of the reach of children, preferably in a locked cabinet.

When children are old enough to understand, warn them about harmful substances. Let them help you affix "Mr. Yuk" labels to bottles and cans containing toxic materials, and teach them that "Mr. Yuk" means Do not touch, Do not smell, Do not taste. Find out the phone number of the nearest poison-control center and keep it near your telephones.

For many years, doctors have suggested that every family with small children keep a bottle of ipecac in the medicine cabinet. It does not require a prescription and is used to induce vomiting. Some doctors and poison-control centers suggest that in addition to ipecac syrup, activated charcoal also be kept. (Of course, this is not the charcoal that you use in your barbecue grill!) Activated charcoal is a substance that can absorb many times its weight in contaminants and has been used for years in Belgium and France as a first line of defense against poisons, but it has not been widely available in the United States.

Please keep in mind that neither of the above remedies should be used until after talking with your doctor or poison-control center. When you find your child playing with a bottle of medicine or cleanser and some of the contents has spilled or is gone, do not presume that your child did not take any of the contents. Always call and get information on what to watch for and what to do. Have the bottle with you when you call so you can supply needed technical information, the possible amount taken, when it occurred, and the current condition of your child. Check for pupil size, lethargy, irritability, flushing, and breathing difficulties. Save any of the remaining ingested substance, and if the child does vomit, save that for possible testing as well. If you are told to seek medical assistance, contact your doctor or emergency room promptly.

According to a toxologist at the Rocky Mountain Poison Center in Denver, Colorado, there is a new superactivated product, called SuperChar Liquid, which has two to three times the absorptive capacity of ordinary activated charcoal.

Q Now that most paints are lead-free, is lead poisoning still a problem a parent needs to be concerned about?

A It's hard to believe that lead poisoning can still be a problem, but it occurs more frequently that one might suspect. Whenever newspapers are burned in a fireplace, lead is released from the print into the environment. As a person sews lead weights into draperies to make them hang straight, care must be taken that small children not get the weights and put them into their mouths. If a weight were swallowed and not removed promptly from the stomach, the resulting lead poisoning could be fatal.

House paint is still a common source of lead poisoning in older neighborhoods. If you live in a pre-World War II home, it's a good idea to remove a paint chip about the size of a quarter and have it analyzed for lead. Please take extreme caution when remodeling, since sanding or scraping this paint will enhance absorption.

Don't let children eat even the cleanest-looking snow, especially in cities or near highways. Lead from air pollution can contaminate the snow.

If you drink soft water from a lead-lined cistern or if you suspect you have old lead plumbing in your home, it's a good idea to take a water sample to the local board of health lab to have it tested for lead content. Soft water is more acidic and absorbs lead more quickly.

Recent evidence suggests that 4 percent of the children between the ages of one and five show increased lead absorption. Children easily absorb lead from their intestines into their bloodstreams. Dietary deficiencies of protein and minerals, excesses of fats and oils increase lead absorption and toxicity.

Adults can also experience lead poisoning. Strong dishwasher soaps can remove the glaze on some pottery and expose a hazardous lead glaze. The elevated lead levels in the blood of garage workers, policemen, and street workers can be traced to the leaded gasoline used in older automobiles. And lead has even been found leaking into acidic pickles from old canning lids. Don't leave acid foods in containers (unless they are glass or plastic) after they have been opened. A recent study showed that lead levels in orange juice increased about seven times when stored in the original cans over a five-day period.

The results of lead poisoning? In children, large amounts of lead in the blood can lead to convulsions, brain damage, or death. Lesser amounts can cause learning disabilities and mental disorders.

In adults, long-term high lead levels are thought to be related to kidney damage leading to subsequent failure, hypertension, loss of reflexes, and slow reaction time caused by damage to nerve fibers.

Q   Should I have my child screened for lead poisoning?

A   The American Academy of Pediatrics (AAP) has stated that, ideally, all preschool children should be screened for lead absorption because exposure to excess lead is widespread and may cause irreversible impairments in children. Certainly children ages one to three years, living in older houses in designated high-risk areas, should be screened. Often there are no symptoms prior to the onset of harmful effects, which range from anemia and behavioral disorders to mental retardation, nerve damage, and even death. Excessive levels of lead also contribute to higher risk of complications in pregnancy.

Although danger of lead poisoning from old peeling paint chips has been widely publicized, a more recent concern is tap water that contains toxic levels of lead. The EPA (Environmental Protection Agency) recently reported that nearly two out of ten Americans consume excessive amounts of lead from their drinking water. Although the public water supplies have very low lead levels, lead from lead joints and soldered pipes leaches into the water supply where it is both colorless and tasteless.

You can curtail lead consumption by running the water for several minutes before using it for cooking or drinking. Contact your local health department for individual water testing and for more information on this subject.

Q   My two year old recently ate a berry from a Jerusalem cherry plant at a friend's house. Luckily we made it through this frightening experience with the help of our poison-control center. Could you list some other common household plants that are poisonous?

A   Besides the berries of the Jerusalem cherry, poisonous holiday plants include poinsettia, mistletoe, English holly. The bulbs of the amaryllis, narcissus, tube rose, and daffodil flowers are also particularly toxic.

Some other poisonous hosehold plants include the following:

asparagus plant
caladium
castor bean
dieffenbachia (dumb cane)
English ivy
philodendron
jequirity bean (one pea chewed will kill an adult)
oleander
evergreen
foxglove
lily of the valley

Plants unlikely to cause toxic reactions from handling or eating include the following:

African violet
baby tears
begonia
Boston fern
Christmas cactus
coleus
corn plant
crab apple
dandelion
dogwood
donkey tail

dracaena
gardenia
grape ivy
hedge apple
honeysuckle
hoya
jade plant
kalanchoe
lily (day, Easter, and tiger)
marigold
Norfolk Island pine
petunia
prayer plant
purple passion
spider plant
Swedish ivy
umbrella violet
wandering Jew
weeping willow
wild onion
zebra plant

All plants should be kept out of the reach of young children, even nontoxic ones, because the child may choke if the plant material becomes caught in his throat.

BURN PREVENTION

Q My neighbor has lowered the temperature of her water heater to prevent burning her children. Is it really that helpful?

A Indeed it is! You can save money and prevent injuries at the same time. Children's sensitive skin, thinner than adults', makes them more vulnerable to burns. Tapwater burns send about 2,500 children to hospital emergency rooms each year. If you have young children in your home, the thermostat of your water heater should be set below 125°F. A small child can suffer a third-degree burn in six seconds when the water is 140° F, but it takes two full minutes for skin to be burned at 125°F. Always keep bathwater lukewarm, testing it yourself before having your child climb in, and never leave a child under the age of four alone in the tub.

CHEMICAL CONTACT WITH EYES

Q   What type of care do you recommend for children who get any kind of chemical in their eyes?

A   Immediately flood the eye with water, either by holding the child's face under gently running tap water, as in the shower, or by gently pouring lukewarm water from a pitcher or glass into the child's eye while he or she is lying down. It is important to hold the eyelid open during the process and to continue the rinsing for at least fifteen minutes. Do not use an eyecup or bandage the eye.

After you have followed these instructions, call the family doctor or poison-control center for any further instructions. Take your child to the doctor quickly if his or her vision is blurred, if there is any mark or cloudy spot on the child's eyes, if the eyes continue to tear or blink, or if the chemical was an acid or alkali. If you are unable to adequately flush the eye, seek medical attention promptly, and take the chemical's container with you.

CHOKING

Q   What are some precautions a parent can take to prevent a choking accident?

A   Choking is the seventh leading cause of accidental pediatric death in the United States, claiming more than 1,300 victims each year. Many of these children choke on food such as hot dogs, candy, nuts, and grapes, which cause more than 40 percent of the deaths.

Adults can take some precautions to safeguard youngsters. Never give nuts, popcorn, or rounded candies to children younger than four years old. Cut grapes and other round, pliable foods into small pieces.

Most people are aware of the danger of small, loose items such as buttons or coins, but are perhaps not aware that disk batteries and miniature batteries used in calculators, cameras, or hearing aids, are also dangerous. Not only can batteries cause children to choke but they also can leak caustic solutions that cause dangerous burns if they lodge in the esophagus.

If you have never learned the "Heimlich Hug," take the time to read about this technique in one of the many pamphlets available. Since Dr. Henry J. Heimlich first introduced the technique in 1974, the lives of several thousand people have been saved.

The following suggestions from Dr. Henry Heimlich were written in response to a teen-age babysitter who requested information about using the Heimlich maneuver on young children who are choking. These tips appeared in the October 1986 edition of *Turtle* magazine, a health publication for children and their parents.

"First of all, I want to remind all teen-agers who babysit what the signs of choking are. A choking child cannot breathe or speak. If an otherwise healthy child suddenly becomes unconscious, is not breathing, and shows no signs of injury, the child is probably a victim of choking.

"*Do not* reach down the child's throat with your fingers and *do not* hit on the back. Either method could force the object down farther into the child's throat and would not save him. *Do not* turn the child upside down, as that can cause an object that was only partially blocking the airway to block it completely.

"The correct procedure for a choking child over the age of two is to reach around from behind the child's back, place one fist against the child's abdomen just above the belly button and cover your fist with your other hand, then press inward and upward quickly.

"After one or two presses, the object should come flying out of the child's mouth. If it doesn't, try again and again. The important thing is not to give up. Meanwhile, shout for help. By the time an adult comes, the incident might be over and the child could be playing again.

"The Heimlich maneuver is not a game; it is a very serious lifesaving method. Practice it on a doll, not on a child. Learn it correctly from a class or a teaching film. To save a life, perform the Heimlich maneuver very gently, especially on a child, or you can cause severe injury. Be absolutely certain that the child is choking or you may cause harm needlessly."

Q   What is the best way to help someone who is choking? At what point should I begin to take some action?

A   For years medical opinion has differed on the best method for dislodging a foreign object from a choking victim. However, at a conference held in July 1985 to establish first-aid standards for the American Red Cross and the American Heart Institute, the participants concluded that only the Heimlich maneuver should be used to relieve a choking victim.

Signs to determine whether a person is choking are 1) the victim cannot speak or breathe; 2) the victim is turning blue; and 3) the victim collapses.

The success of the Heimlich maneuver lies in the fact that a person has a large volume of air in his lungs. This reservoir of air is expelled when a rescuer presses sharply and repeatedly on the victim's abdomen with a balled fist grasped by the opposite hand, at a point just above the navel and below the rib cage. The force of the air being pushed from the lungs will dislodge the obstruction from the throat.

Q What procedure should you use first for a drowning victim—the Heimlich maneuver or CPR?

A The National Conference on Standards and Guidelines for Cardiopulmonary Resuscitation and Emergency Cardiac Care has now endorsed the abdominal thrusts of the Heimlich maneuver as the first step in treating drowning victims. Heretofore, the advice had been to remove any foreign object from the victim's mouth and then begin mouth-to-mouth resuscitation.

Though the principle is the same as that used on choking victims, the maneuver is applied to drowning victims in a flat rather than in a standing position.

Place the drowning victim on his back, remove any foreign objects from his mouth, and turn his head to one side. Then straddle the victim's thighs and place both of your fists firmly on the person's upper stomach at the edge of the rib cage. With a quick upward motion, push the fists under the rib cage and into the diaphragm. This could expel a considerable quantity of water, but you can apply a second maneuver to expel any remaining water. Dr. Heimlich recommended that this measure be employed first in attempting to resuscitate drowning victims, because "you have to get the water out of the lungs before you can get the air in."

The victim should begin to breathe at this point, but if not, begin mouth-to-mouth resuscitation.

HYPOTHERMIA

Q How long can a person survive under water? What treatment should be given for hypothermia?

A Not long ago physicians and rescue workers were taught that irreversible damage occurred to the brain after four minutes without oxygen and death after six minutes. However, Dr. Martin Nemiroff, an authority on hypothermia and a member of the Great Lakes U. S. Coast Guard, witnessed the survival of a girl who was submerged for seventy minutes in cold Alaskan water. Dr. Nemiroff says young children in particular have a good chance of surviving in cold waters.

Many hypothermic people appear as though they are dead after being in water or exposed to cold temperatures. Their pulse may be undetectable and their skin blue, but they are still alive. While the body's surface temperature may be greatly reduced, the core temperature may be warmer and the circulation altered, thus protecting the heart, lungs, and other vital organs. Symptoms of milder hypothermia include drowsiness, slurred speech, euphoria, and inability to feel the cold. Mental confusion often prevents the victim from thinking clearly about survival.

When most of us think of situations leading to hypothermia, we envision temperatures of 40 to 60 degrees below zero. Yet far more cases of fatal hypothermia occur in rainy 40-degree weather. Being wet and cold is worse than suffering from the cold alone. Most people prepare for the dramatic cold temperatures, but may be very casual about the cool, damp days that pose such a problem to maintaining body temperatures.

When a person is submerged in cold water, the water robs the body of its heat much more quickly than does air. Thus, if a person clings to a boat or life jacket, he or she should try to stay as far out of the water as possible to increase chances of survival. Another technique to conserve body heat in water is to huddle with other survivors, which increases survival chances.

A moderate to severely hypothermic person must be rewarmed under controlled circumstances. Otherwise the cold and stagnated blood may suddenly return to the heart and other vital organs, possibly causing a heart attack and death just as resuscitation begins.

TRAVEL TIPS

Q The national news recently reported a study showing that rear-seat lap belts did more harm than good. My preschoolers no longer use car seats. Should we continue to use rear-seat lap belts?

A The answer is an emphatic yes! Diane K. Steed, administrator of the National Highway Traffic Safety Administration (NHTSA), issued a statement concerning the National Traffic Safety Board's (NTSB) study on lap belts. She stated that the study was based on an extremely small data base that does not give a true picture of safety-belt performance. The study looked only at frontal crashes, in which rear-seat lap belts are particularly ineffective. They also looked at injuries caused by the belts and ignored situations such as ejections, which are generally fatal and are prevented by belt usage.

The NHTSA studied thousands of cases and clearly showed that a person riding in the back seat has a much better chance of avoiding serious injury or death if that person is wearing a safety belt. However, usage of a shoulder-lap belt, when available, is recommended over a lap belt alone.

Motor vehicle crashes are the leading cause of death for children one to fifteen years of age. They are also the number 1 *preventable* cause of children's deaths. Parental use of seat belts greatly influences their children's decisions to wear their seat belts. *Please buckle up!*

Q My wife and I have planned a trip around the world. What health tips can you offer to ensure that we'll enjoy our time in a foreign country?

A A dream vacation to a foreign country can turn out to be a nightmare if you are unprepared for a medical emergency.

Vaccinations for foreign travel are usually the first step

in preparing for your vacation. Check with your local or state board of health for vaccination requirements for the countries being visited. Take all vaccination records with you.

No vaccination is available for malaria. However, medication taken before, during, and after travel defends against this illness. With an estimated 200 to 400 million malaria cases reported annually world-wide, you should carefully consider this precaution in your travel plans. Ask your travel agent and local health department about countries with a high rate of malaria.

Those traveling to central African countries should be aware of the AIDS-infected blood supply there. See the chapter on AIDS for precautions. Those traveling to Ethiopia should be aware of louse-born typhus in that country. There is no vaccine for it, but doxycycline for treating it can be carried in the event the symptoms occur.

Probably the most common travelers' complaint is diarrhea. Though uncomfortable and inconvenient, it is the body's way of sloughing off noxious agents. The major medical complications from diarrhea are dehydration and electrolyte imbalance. Unchlorinated water, contaminated fruits and vegetables, raw fish or undercooked meats can bring on such a bout. An eight-ounce glass of bottled orange or apple juice with one-half teaspoon of corn syrup and a pinch of salt, followed by eight ounces of boiled or carbonated water with one-quarter teaspoon of baking soda stirred in will help to restore the body's water and electrolyte balance.

Packing a bottle or two of an over-the-counter anti-diarrhea medicine can ensure a much more pleasant vacation. Your doctor may suggest a preventive medication regime.

A well-packed first-aid kit should also be on your list and should include the following:

- antiseptic ointment for burns or cuts
- nasal decongestants

- motion-sickness medication
- water-purification tablets
- Band-Aids
- tweezers
- gauze pads
- aspirin or aspirin substitutes
- antacids
- calamine lotion
- insect repellent
- thermometer

Carrying an extra pair of prescription glasses is a good idea, as is carrying a statement indicating major health problems you may have and any medications you are taking or may need. Of course, don't forget to wear any necessary medical I.D. bracelets or tags. Regular medications, such as insulin, should be carried with you rather than being packed in baggage that could be lost or delayed.

If you are prone to motion sickness, sit over the wings or as close as possible to them when flying.

While flying, passengers often consume more than their usual amount of alcohol because of its availability and because the dryness of the airplane cabin may increase thirst. Ross McFarland, professor of Aerospace Health and Safety at Harvard, warns that alcohol is 33 percent more potent at usual cruise altitudes than at sea level. Because of the decreased atmospheric pressure, alcohol reaches the blood faster than usual. Thus, reduce your intake to less than your usual amount.

SAFE SUNNING

Q   Just how safe are tanning booths? I see people on my college campus with dark tans in the middle of winter. Are these artificial rays doing more harm than good?

A   Tanning salons began almost a decade ago when a real-estate broker opened the first salon in Searcy, Arkansas. Now there are thousands of salons in operation in all fifty states.

Minutes in a tanning booth are equivalent to hours in the sun minus the heat, sweat, and sand. However, the ultraviolet rays can result in future skin problems. Researchers report that a sun lamp can produce nearly seven times more DNA damage per unit of reddened skin than the sun. And dermatologists almost universally oppose the use of tanning salons.

Other hazards that are not immediately obvious are skin and eye sensitivities. People with a photosensitivity disease, such as lupus erythematosus, could be harmed by using a booth. Lupus is a disease of unknown cause that produces skin lesions on the face, neck, and extremities. Persons with vitiligo, those white patches on the skin due to the absence of pigment, should also stay clear of the UV lights. Medications, such as chloroquin and tetracycline, cause photosensitivity, which means that certain individuals could get a severe allergic reaction if taking any of these drugs while subjecting themselves to the UV rays.

In short, avoid the booths.

It would most likely prove a wasted effort to try to persuade the public to abandon the world of fun in the sun, so the next best move is to educate the public in the use of sunscreens. Sunscreens come with an SPF number, which indicates the effectiveness of blocking the sun's rays. Doctors recommend the sunscreens rated "15," because that means it takes fifteen times as long to get a sunburn with the sunscreen as without it.

Screening out the sun's UV rays isn't just to prevent wrinkling. Basal cell skin cancer commonly results from excessive exposure to harmful sun rays. Skin cancer, rarely a problem before 1930, is now prevalent. It develops primarily on those areas of the skin excessively exposed to the sun—face, neck, arms, hands, legs, back. With appropriate treatment this cancer can easily be cured, but don't delay in seeking help.

Of course, not all sun exposure is bad. Dr. D. M. Davies of London stated that lack of sunlight for two to three weeks can begin to deplete the body's vitamin D level enough to cause inadequate intestinal absorption of calcium. Dr. Robert M. Neer of Massachusetts General Hospital commented that elderly people would benefit by getting outside more during daylight hours. In addition to the physiologic importance of sunlight, light also positively affects mood and behavior.

ELECTRICAL SHOCK

Q   What should a person do to prevent electrical shock? Does a person act as a conductor for an electrical current?

A   Benjamin Franklin was lucky: his famous electrical experiment could have killed him. According to the National Safety Council, approximately 1,000 people die every year in electrical accidents with 10 percent of those occurring in the home.

Electrical pressure, or voltage, pushes the current of electrons along the circuit like water through a pipe. It's dangerous only when a person becomes part of that circuit. One of the major risks in the home is between the wall outlet and an appliance or a lamp. For instance, when wires are run underneath rugs or furniture, the insulation can wear thin and leave bare wires. This condition may lead to the twin dangers of shock and fire.

Also, leaving a lightbulb socket empty can have tragic consequences for someone putting a finger in by mistake. Wall outlets should be covered with plastic inserts so that inquisitive toddlers don't stick their fingers or other objects into them.

Avoid holding electrical appliances near water. Make sure you don't place curlers, hot combs, or hair dryers near a tub or shower for them to fall in. If they should fall into the water when plugged in, they can electrocute you even if they are not turned on.

In the kitchen, take care when cleaning cooking appliances such as crock pots and waffle irons that aren't labeled "immersible." If you place them in the sink to clean them, moisture clings to the inside and can cause a shock the next time they are used.

All major appliances, such as stoves and refrigerators, should be grounded using a three-prong outlet and plug. If the appliance has a three-prong plug, but your home still has two-prong outlets, do *not* cut off the ground. Instead, go to the hardware store and get a three-prong converter. Be sure to attach the extra wire of the adapter to the screw in the center of the outlet's face plate to ground it.

Use extreme caution when the basement floods. If the water level is above the motors of electrical equipment, call the utility company to shut off the power. Qualified repair persons should check everything in the basement before the power is turned back on.

When you approach downed wires after a storm, whether or not they are sparking, remember to stay out of water puddles and damp grass. Electricity can travel many feet through puddles and cause shock injuries. If you are in an automobile accident that has caused utility wires to fall to the ground and you're inside the car, stay there. The rubber tires will insulate the car. Don't touch any metal objects, and wait for help to arrive.

Make sure that an electrical-shock victim is breathing and has a heartbeat. Keep the victim warm and elevate his or her feet to ward off circulatory shock and to increase blood flow to the brain. If you see no chest movement, hear no breathing sounds, and feel no pulse, begin CPR (cardiopulmonary resuscitation) immediately and call for help.

Would you know how to perform CPR? If not, call a local hospital or the American Red Cross for information about classes providing CPR instruction. The course involves a very short time commitment but could help you save a life.

RADON HAZARD

Q   Articles on radon appear frequently in our local newspaper. What are the effects of this natural hazard? Should we have our house tested even though we live in a new house in the open country?

A   Yes, it's a good idea to have your home tested. The U. S. Environmental Protection Agency and the Centers for Disease Control are concerned about the increased risk of developing lung cancer faced by persons exposed to above-average levels of radon in their homes. Radon, a naturally occurring radioactive gas, is believed to cause 13,000 lung-cancer deaths per year in the United States and is believed to be the leading cause of lung-cancer deaths in nonsmokers.

My sister, who neither smoked nor lived or worked with anyone who smoked, had surgery for lung cancer. The basement of her house showed radon levels at more than twice the acceptable levels. We don't know if that was the cause, but a professor from Cornell University, who tested forty homes in the Des Moines, Iowa, area where my sister lives, found that 30 percent had dangerously high levels of radon. This odorless, colorless, and tasteless gas could contaminate as many as 8 million homes in America, according to the EPA. The age of the home makes little difference; in fact, new homes, because of their airtight building structure, may be more prone to have a radon problem.

Radon has been detected in significant amounts in nearly every state in the nation. But levels of radon gas found out-of-doors are not harmful, because radon concentrations are low. Your risk of developing lung cancer from exposure to radon is largely dependent on the concentrations of the gas in your home and the length of time you're exposed to it. Homes in areas where radon is emitted by the earth tend to concentrate the gas, making it potentially lethal.

Radon gas is measured in units called picocuries per liter. The EPA recently announced that as many as one out of eight homes in America may exceed the four picocuries per liter the EPA has set as the action level for radon exposure.

How do you find out if your home contains radon? We checked sources of radon testers and found one fairly simple and inexpensive method, which is an activated charcoal type that resembles a huge tea bag. Open the bag and leave it in your home for three days; then send it to an EPA-approved laboratory for analysis. The lab will return your test results within twenty-four hours after receiving the detector. (The lab charges a nominal fee for reading the test and mailing the results.)

Radon contamination can be reduced to acceptable levels by sealing the radon's entry points and circulating more outside air into your home. Radon gas can move through small spaces in the soil and rock and enter the house through cracks in the concrete, sump pumps, joints, and floor drains.

There are some easy ways to reduce your risk of radon exposure. Discourage any smoking in your house (smoking increases the hazardous effect of radon exposure). Spend less time in areas with higher radon concentrations, such as the basement. And when practical, open windows and turn on fans to increase the outside airflow into the house, which helps to dilute the radon concentration inside. If you have a crawl space, keep the vents open year-round.

Contact your nearest regional EPA office or state radiation-protection office for test information.

Index